# HOSPITAL
## Survival Guide

Dr. David Sherer's

# HOSPITAL
## Survival Guide

**100+** Ways to Make Your Hospital Stay Safe and Comfortable

BY DAVID SHERER, MD AND MARYANN KARINCH

Dr. David Sherer's Hospital Survival Guide
100+ Ways to Make Your Hospital Stay Safe and Comfortable

David Sherer, M.D., and Maryann Karinch

Published by Claren Books
A Division of Adler & Robin Books, Inc.
   3000 Connecticut Avenue, N.W.
   Washington, D.C. 20008
   adlerbooks@adlerbooks.com
   http://www.adlerbooks.com
   http://www.clarenbooks.com

Printed in the United States of America. First Edition

Library of Congress Cataloging-in-Publication Data

Sherer, David.
   Dr. David Sherer's hospital survival guide : 100+ ways to make your
hospital stay safe and comfortable / by David Sherer and Maryann Karinch.
        p. cm.
Includes bibliographical references and index.
   ISBN 0-9723736-0-8 (pbk.)
   1. Hospital care—Popular works.  2. Hospital patients—Popular works.
3. Consumer education—Popular works.  I. Title: Doctor David Sherer's
hospital survival guide.  II. Title: Hospital survival guide.  III. Karinch, Maryann.
IV. Title.
   RA965.6.S53 2003
   362.1'1—dc21
                                                2003008931
                                                    CIP

# DEDICATION

For *Laura* and *Liam*

For *Dr. Ronald L. Kotler,*
who embodies everything good about being a doctor

For my father, *Dr. Max G. Sherer,*
healer, humorist, intellect, and golfer

In honor of the memory of my sister,
*Lisa Beth Sherer*

# CONTENTS

The "100+ Ways" are in **boldface** throughout the book. Key terms and concepts in the text that are defined in the Glossary are *italicized* when first introduced.

| | | |
|---|---|---|
| INTRODUCTION | How This Book Can Help Make Your Hospital Stay Safe and Comfortable | 1 |
| CHAPTER 1 | You've Just Found Out You Need Surgery— Now What? | 5 |
| CHAPTER 2 | Choosing the Best Hospital for Safety and Comfort | 27 |
| CHAPTER 3 | The Pre-surgery Interview: What Every Patient Needs to Know | 43 |
| CHAPTER 4 | All About Anesthesia: How to Make Sure Your Doctor Knows What It Takes to Keep You Out of Pain | 71 |
| CHAPTER 5 | Taking Care of Business: Insurance, Advance Heath Care Directives, Wills and Other Matters | 95 |
| CHAPTER 6 | Getting Ready to Go: Packing and Other Practical Details | 115 |
| CHAPTER 7 | In the Hospital | 137 |
| CHAPTER 8 | When Your Child Has to Go to the Hospital | 165 |
| CHAPTER 9 | When You Have No Time to Plan: Advice for Emergency Room Patients | 177 |
| CHAPTER 10 | Working the System to Get What You Need | 205 |
| CHAPTER 11 | Leaving the Hospital ... and Beyond | 241 |

APPENDIX **A**     Sample Emergency Medical ID Card          257

APPENDIX **B**     Common Outpatient (Same Day) Procedures   259

APPENDIX **C**     Hospital Jargon: A Sample Dialog
                   (with Translation)                       269

APPENDIX **D**     Useful Websites                           273

APPENDIX **E**     Glossary of Hospital Terms                281


**A**CKNOWLEDGMENTS                                          299

**I**NDEX                                                    301

**A**BOUT THE **A**UTHORS                                    311

# How This Book Can Help
# Make Your Hospital Stay
# Safe and Comfortable

When I first went on a roller coaster, my friends had to drag me into the car. They wanted me to ride the Thunderbolt in Pittsburgh with them, and I had no idea what to expect. As the cars started tracking up and kept going higher and higher, I said to my friend next to me, "They have to stop this thing because I'm getting off!" My fear of heights ratcheted up a notch with each click of the cars inching their way to the top of the first hill. My friend said, "They can't stop it." I said, "They're gonna stop it—now!" I felt overwhelmed and out of control. I went into the ride totally ignorant, and my worst fears were realized. Sure, I made it through, but it was *not* a pleasant experience.

When you enter the hospital as a patient, many strange sights, sounds, and sensations can ratchet up your fear in a similar way. And you have much less choice than I did about the roller-coaster ride— plus more important questions about what the experience will involve. Fear of the unknown is, of course, perfectly normal. A hospital stay is replete with unknowns, and you can't just dismiss your concerns or criticize yourself if the thought of going to the hospital frightens you— even a little.

This book will help you know how far you're going to go up, when you zig, when you zag, and how your stomach will feel when you're upside down, so you will face fewer unknowns on the hospital "thrill ride."

To determine what information to put in this book, I looked back at a lifetime of exposure to medical issues and nearly twenty years of my own interaction with patients. By "lifetime" I mean the years before medical school, when I learned about patient concerns from my dad, a doctor, and my mom, a nurse. When I was a kid, I used to go on rounds with my dad, who is still a practicing physician in his eighties. I saw how scared and uncomfortable people could be. Another important person who fueled my desire to help patients feel safer and more comfortable was my sister, whose frequent complications from severe diabetes made her a revolving-door hospital patient for much of her all-too-brief life.

In short, the impetus to write this book sprang from a broad range of personal relationships and personal experiences. There was no triggering incident, no particular horror story, that's behind it. It's just my family background and the day-to-day experience I have as a doctor seeing patients who are scared and uncomfortable: patients who desperately want to regain some control over their lives.

As an anesthesiologist, I commonly see patients at the height of their confusion and sense of helplessness. My presence reminds them that surgery is imminent, an awareness that often shocks them into asking questions.

I come to meet you after you've put on the hospital gown that leaves private parts exposed and after you've been given that hideous "shower cap" to cover your hair. All of a sudden you realize: "This is for real—I'm going to be unconscious in a room full of strangers and gadgets." All of a sudden, you crave the details of your impending experience and wish you knew if anything can be done to make it better.

Every day before I administer anesthesia, I hear a stream of "what ifs?" and "then whats?" The trouble is, most of the questions I get at this point ought to have been answered far earlier in the process. The answers and reassurances should have come from the patients' own primary care physicians, or from specialists, or from the nursing staff, or from hospital administrators or from the health insurance company. Because I may not have the needed answers, the patient ends up going into surgery feeling more anxious than ever.

That shouldn't happen. Every patient has a right to know what's going to go on when something is about to be done to his or her body—and beyond that, what your recovery period is going to be like while you're in the hospital and what are your long-term prospects for recovery. In this book you will find out how to get that information from the right source and at the right time—as well as what to do if you receive unsatisfactory or unintelligible answers.

From the beginning to the end of your hospital experience, you have a right to expect professional people at the hospital to respect you and respond to your needs in a professional manner. There's a flip side to your expectations, though. The hospital staff has a right to expect you to be open and honest about your condition and reasonable about the things you want done for your comfort. They will expect you to be calm and cooperative, at least to the extent that you can manage it, while you are being poked and interrogated. They realize that waking you up at four o'clock in the morning may turn you into a crank; you realize that they're not just waking you up out of a sadistic desire to deprive you of sleep, but because there is some clear medical purpose for doing so that can't be postponed. (If, however, they are waking you for a reason that could well be postponed, this book will tell you how to get them to do it!)

To help you make your hospital stay safe and comfortable, this book will address the most common patient questions and problems, plus many others you may not have thought of. I will alert you to potentially deadly mistakes, but also point out some of the small but annoying things about hospital care that you can learn to avoid, once you're in the know. I will also tell you stories of real people and their experiences (although I have changed names and other identifying information for those individuals who requested anonymity). All in all, this book will be your insider's guide to make the hospital system work for you, so that you can enjoy (all right, "enjoy" is probably an overstatement) the safest and most comfortable hospital stay possible.

*David Sherer, M.D.*

# CHAPTER 1

# You've Just Found Out You Need Surgery—Now What?

In this chapter you will learn

- A few important things *not* to do before or during your hospital stay
- How to find a surgeon you can trust with your body and your life
- How to find out if you really need the operation you've been told you should have
- How and why to get a second opinion

**Avoid having elective surgery in July.**
I'm beginning with this tip because it's an easy mistake to avoid, if you're having the sort of surgery that can be planned some time in advance. The discussion that follows explains why July is the worst month to be in the hospital:

The academic calendar for medical schools includes an entry like this at the beginning of July:

> 3rd Year Mandatory Orientation/Registration
> Introduction to Clinical Skills

That means medical students who have made it through courses like anatomy, pharmacology, and medical ethics finally get experience with patients. If you are one of those patients and you are in a *university,* or *university-affiliated,* hospital, you will see old medical teams vanish and new ones take over. It's the *July syndrome:* Interns, residents, and graduating medical students who have finished their training at that hospital leave, and fresh faces appear in the operating room, on the wards, and at your bedside.

When I was training, I heard the attending senior physicians say things like, "Here we go with another July. I have to take my nerve medicine." I had an anesthesia professor who said he'd have a nervous breakdown every July trying to make sure the neophytes didn't hurt anybody.

On a positive note, if you are in a university hospital in July, you have the energy and curiosity of people who have dreamed of this moment for years. They may be more interested in the academic aspect of your problem than more jaded doctors. They may talk with you more. They may share articles on your problem with you. At least, that's how I'd advise you to look at your situation if your July surgery absolutely cannot be rescheduled.

But if you can avoid having raw novices learning on your body, then by all means do so. Even the brightest and most dedicated medical students will make a few mistakes in the beginning—although they are theoretically under a doctor's supervision at all times.

When my friend Dennis was just entering his third year of medical school, he was learning to draw blood. He wasn't very good at it, but he finally succeeded with his first patient after several sticks. Back at the nursing station, he soon found out he had put the blood in the wrong tube. "Go back and draw some more," the intern told him. Dennis didn't want to go back to he patient and admit he'd done the wrong thing, so he said, "Mr. Jones, we need an additional, special test besides the original test. Did I mention that to you?"

"Oh, no! Do I have to go through this again?" the patient moaned.

"I'm sorry, your attending doctor ordered this," Dennis lied, as he prepared the unsuspecting man for a fresh jab.

The poor patient in this case had no idea that he was Dennis's first blood draw. But if you find yourself in a hospital in July and you see a young person hovering over you nervously with a needle, you are hereby warned that you, too, could be in for the pincushion treatment. Which brings me to my next, and also extremely important tip:

## Stand on your right not to be a medical student's guinea pig.

The patients' empowerment movement has led to some much needed reforms in hospitals—chiefly, the creation in many hospitals of an office of patient advocacy (more about this in Chapter 5)—but one right that every patient has and should insist upon is the right to refuse treatment from someone whose skills appear uncertain. The next tip contains some further advice on that point.

## Find out how experienced your caregivers are.

The trouble is, you may not be sure if the person sticking you with the needle is good at her job or not. If that's the case, you will need to ask a blunt question or two. Ask: "How long have you been doing this?"

But don't expect anyone to admit, "You're my first." You'll probably get some kind of vague reassurance: "Oh, I've had lots of practice in the lab." Just remember: That could mean on lab rats ... or even oranges. Unless you get a confident response along the lines of "I've done hundreds of patients and I've been told I'm especially good with hard-to-find veins," you should have no hesitation about going to the next tip.

## Call for a nurse or lab technician to take over.

If you don't get a specific answer that satisfies you as to the person's competence (say, three months at a minimum, or half a year, to allow for the fact that some students require a longer learning curve), you can and should say, "Wait. I think I would like to have the nurse do this." You need not apologize or feel defensive about your request. It's your body and protecting yourself in the hospital from inexperienced staff members is more important than giving a medical student an opportunity to perfect her skills.

Let the medical student learn on someone who hasn't read this book.

## Know who the decision-makers are in the crowd.

Another July syndrome problem: With a host of new medical students on board, you must expect to be examined and quizzed more than usual, and you may be confused by the appearance of so many new people in white coats. Should you feel obligated to repeat your medical history to everyone? Who among all these young faces is making recommendations on your care? In mid-summer, these are serious concerns for the patient in a teaching hospital.

You might want to learn right now what you can do to tell who's who and figure out where each person fits in the hospital chain of command. If that's your strategy, go right to Chapter 10, "Working the System to Get What You Need." But it's so much simpler in most cases to avoid the situation altogether by staying away from any teaching or university hospital in July (except, of course, in the case of a medical emergency).

## Avoid scheduling major elective surgery for late in the day.

This is another simple thing you should know right from the start: You should schedule your surgery for the morning, for safety as well as a convenience reasons, if you have any choice in the matter.

Like anyone else who is expending mental and physical energy on the job, doctors and nurses can become fatigued late in the day. In a report aired on the *NBC Nightly News* on August 15, 2001, hospital staff fatigue was cited as one of the most common reasons for errors in anesthesia administration. Patients who were scheduled third, fourth, or even later for anesthesia were markedly more likely to be the victims of careless mistakes.

Also consider that most operating room teams change shift around three o'clock in the afternoon; if you're an afternoon surgery patient, you won't have the same continuity of care that you'd have as a morning patient. The problems that arise from the shift change are similar to those caused by the July syndrome above, but on a daily basis.

Consider this scenario: During your afternoon surgery, there's a complication of some sort. The staff who have to cope with the complication are not only tired but anxious to leave—but now, because of you, they'll be leaving late. Do you really want people working on you who might resent the fact that they'll miss their child's soccer game? Or if they don't get out the door in the next ten minutes, they won't be able to use the freeway that becomes carpool-only usage at rush hour?

Then there's your own comfort to consider: Your pre-surgery instructions almost certainly will ban you from putting anything in your mouth during the eight hours before surgery. With morning surgery that's not much of a problem because you sleep all night; the only meal you have to skip is breakfast. But depriving yourself of both breakfast and lunch and, perhaps, an afternoon snack as well, is a much tougher thing to do.

And it's not like you can get a normal half workday in by having your surgery later in the day. You're still going to have to arrive hours early, most likely just to sit around and wait. Meanwhile you'll be nervous and sweaty, but not allowed to shower. They may take your clothes away from you at the start, leaving you in nothing but that awkward and embarrassing hospital gown. Not a good start for your hospital experience.

In Chapters 6 and 7 you'll find tips to make the waiting conditions more tolerable, but let me repeat the main advice of this section, which is to eliminate the daytime waiting whenever possible by choosing to have your procedure done first thing in the morning.

## Pick the best surgeon you can get.

Without a doubt, your most important choice as far as safety is concerned is over who is going to be getting inside your body and doing things in there. Obviously, you want the best that's available to you. The tips that follow will help you to find what you're looking for.

But first, you need to find out just how much choice you have. For those in *health maintenance organizations (HMOs),* the answer may be: not much. Your primary care physician does the referral, and the pool of choices is limited to your HMO's list of in-network surgeons. If the best in your area isn't on that list, tough luck.

But that's not to say that you're stuck with the name of whatever random person happens to be available from the list that week. You can and should research the choices, get recommendations, and do all the other things I recommend here for those who have a wide-open choice. You will just have fewer surgeons to compare, that's all. You can and should still pick the best among the names available to you—and then make sure that your primary care physician will affirm your choice by referring you to that surgeon.

### Find a board-certified surgeon.

How do you, the layperson, figure out who's good at a particular operation? You let other medical experts do much of the grading. There is already a process in place to measure how long and how well a surgeon (or any other medical specialist) does what he or she has been trained to do, and that process is called *board certification.*

When a physician has studied a specialty at an advanced level for a number of years, taking and passing required and elective courses, then he or she will be designated "board eligible." At that point, the doctor is permitted to take the board certification examination in his or her specialty or sub-specialty. It's a tough test, let me tell you. Once passed, the doctor is board certified in his or her specialty, patients can feel reassured that that doctor is fully qualified to perform all the standard procedures of that specialty on patients.

How do you find out if your prospective surgeon is board certified? Doctors are not shy about saying so. In fact, any board-certified doctor is bound to plaster that fact on his or her business cards, brochures, and patient information sheets. If you don't see board certification listed, however, you should definitely ask.

If you have a number of doctors under consideration and don't want to call each office, a quick way to find out who's board certified is to go to the Internet and visit the website of the *American Board of Medical Specialties (ABMS)* at ***www.abms.org***. There you will find a free Certified Doctor Verification Service, which will enable you to locate any board-certified physician by city and state, or to search the listings by any of the specialties certified by one or more of the twenty-four Member Boards of the ABMS. All you need is the correct spelling of the physician's name and verification is a click away.

Suppose you find out that your prospective surgeon is not yet board certified but is only board eligible? In that case, it's a good idea to find out if the surgeon is in practice with others who are already board certified. That tells you that other, more experienced hands are happy to have this surgeon on their team. They trust his or her work and have confidence that the doctor has the skills and knowledge to pass the board certification exam when the time comes.

And what if you discover that the person is neither board certified nor board eligible? Frankly, unless your insurance plan ties you to the person, I would say keep looking.

### Collect recommendations from other doctors.

Who knows who's considered good at what in the medical profession? Other doctors do. Patients often come to me and say, "If you were having this knee surgery [or whatever the procedure is], who would you want to do it?" I know lots of doctors in lots of specialties, and frequently I personally know the doctor that I think is the right choice.

In cases where I don't personally know many practitioners in a certain field, I might still know of a few doctors by reputation. Or I might ask around among my colleagues, and be able to pass along a name that several other doctors recommend with confidence.

Your primary care doctor won't mind taking on this job for you. In fact he or she will most likely be pleased that you have come to him or her seeking guidance, and so will probably put a lot of thought and careful judgment into the matter.

### Listen to what other patients have to say.

By now you should have the names of some doctors who are board certified (or board eligible) and accepted by your insurance plan, and from among those you have a name or two recommended by your doctor. Are you done yet? Not quite. It's also quite helpful to get the patient's perspective. After all, your doctor makes recommendations as a colleague, and from somewhat of a distance. Of course, it's a good thing to hear from one doctor that another is highly regarded, but it's even more of a plus to hear from someone who directly benefited from that person's touch. Other patients can tell you things about the doctor that aren't on his or her résumé: Is he good at explaining in lay terms what the procedure entails—or abrupt and cold, throwing a lot of jargon at you? Is she sensitive and patient with those who are nervous, or is she arrogant, dismissive of a patient's fears?

When a fellow patient tells you, "My surgeon was wonderful—not only did she do a great job, but she was terrific at explaining what she was doing every step along the way," that's definitely someone to consider for the job.

To find other patients who might recommend a surgeon, just start asking around among family and friends: Has anyone—even if it's only an acquaintance or a friend of a friend—had the same sort of procedure you are about to undergo? If you get some names of former patients who had a good experience with a surgeon, contact them and find out in detail how it went. If your contact was dissatisfied, see if you can figure out whether the problem stemmed from some quirk of the patient telling the story, or if the fault really belonged to the doctor.

When you hear from other patients as well as from your doctor that a surgeon is great, you can really feel confident in the person you've found.

---

*Bill's back was killing him.* He'd been to his primary care doctor, who suggested physical therapy and other non-surgical treatments. Weeks passed, and the pain kept getting worse. He went back to his primary care doctor, who suggested that Bill ask for an appointment with a neurosurgeon, Dr. Jeffries. Before Bill made the appointment, he decided to see if anyone he knew had another doctor to recommend.

As it happened, Bill's father-in-law had been successfully treated for a similar back problem several years before, and so had his wife's best friend. Bill called each to ask who had done their surgery. Each replied (independently of the other), "Dr. Jeffries"—and each reported being very happy with the results. With two former patients separately telling him how great Dr. Jeffries was, Bill hesitated no further and called for an appointment, which, by the end of the same week, had led to a surgical solution to Bill's back pain.

---

## Find out if the doctor has written articles for medical journals or participated in cutting-edge studies.

Here's a final idea for helping you learn how your prospective surgeon ranks in his or her specialty: Research the doctor's published work. "Cutting-edge" doctors often do more than treat patients; they're involved in research, too, and they publish their results in medical journals like the *New England Journal of Medicine* or the *Journal of the American Medical Association (JAMA),* to name just two of the most prestigious ones.

You may not have the research skills to find out who has written medical journal articles or run studies about the procedure you will be having, but the librarian of any medical library should be able to help you find the information you seek. Running a specific doctor's name through a database of medical authors should take only a second or two, and you will find out what (if any) published research your prospective surgeon has been involved in.

You can also do the research in the other direction: Search for articles or studies about a specific procedure and find out what doctors have written about it or designed studies to evaluate its effectiveness; then find out if one of those doctors might be able to take you on as a patient.

This is especially worth pursuing if the procedure you will be undergoing is new and/or controversial. In that case, you may also want to read articles and study reports by doctors who take the opposing point of view before you make a final choice.

## When it comes to a difficult procedure, give greatest weight to the person with the highest level of skill.

Now, given the choice between someone who is a top expert in his or her field and someone less prominent but having a great "bedside manner" (as reported by former patients), I would probably go with the expert. After all, a medical procedure is usually a one-time thing: You don't really need to develop warm and fuzzy feelings for the person who does it, but you *do* need to be sure that your doctor really knows what he or she is doing. One of the surest signs of such knowledge is to have authored articles or headed studies published in any of the nation's leading medical journals.

**In cases calling for advanced or specialized care, choose a specialist over a generalist who also practices that specialty.**
You're usually better off with a doctor who deals with the particular part of the body or body system that's causing the problem, day in and day out, and who does nothing else in addition.

Let me take as an example a patient who needs to have fibroid tumors removed from her uterus. She could see a general surgeon, a gynecological surgeon (a specialist), or a reproductive surgeon (a gynecological sub-specialist). Suppose this patient's goal, other than getting the tumors out safely, is preserving her reproductive capabilities so that she still has a chance of getting pregnant and carrying a baby to term.

The general surgeon may know a lot about removing benign growths wherever they occur, but he or she isn't focused specifically on female organs. The gynecological surgeon almost certainly will be more familiar with the ins and outs (and possible complications) of surgery on the uterus, but it's the reproductive surgeon whose practice is centered around the preservation and functioning of the reproductive organs. Given a choice among three highly rated surgeons—each considered tops in his or her field—my recommendation in most cases would be to go with the one with the most specialized training in the specific area of the body involved in the procedure.

**Interview the surgeon.**
Once you have the name of a surgeon who comes highly recommended, has got the credentials, and is respected in his or her field, you'll set up an appointment for a consultation. That's the surgeon's opportunity to examine you and figure out the best way to deal with your problem. This examination may well culminate in a recommendation for surgery.

Before you schedule your appointment for this pre-operative consultation, be sure to read Chapter 3, "The Pre-surgery Interview," which is all about the kinds of questions you'll be asked and the kind of information you need to get across to increase your chances of having a safe and successful procedure.

My advice right now, however, is still about being sure you've picked the right sort of person to work with. Use your first meeting with the surgeon as your opportunity to size up this person who may be the one to operate on you. Your face- to-face impression can be as important a factor in your choice as your review of the person's qualifications and background.

To help you discover whether you'll be able to work effectively with this doctor, you should be considering a variety of factors, including some that are more practical than medical in nature, such as: Is the office in a convenient location? Can you get through on the telephone, or do you keep getting lost on endless holds? Is the office well run and professionally staffed? Does the doctor have access to the usual diagnostic equipment, or must you travel to some distant location for the normal run of tests? Then there are some other matters that are harder to put your finger on: Does her manner inspire confidence, or does she seem overly busy and distracted by many interruptions? Is he a good communicator, or does he rush over your test results, not pausing to find out if you understand?

If you find yourself answering more than two or three of the above questions with less than satisfactory responses, you should consider whether you have indeed found the best person to perform your needed procedure. In that case, if you still have the time, it may be wisest to keep looking.

## Consider age and experience.

In your interview with the recommended surgeon, you should ask, "How many operations like mine have you done?" Or "How many years have you been doing this procedure?"

When it comes to surgery, more and longer is almost always better. Studies consistently show that the more experience a doctor has doing a procedure the better the outcomes.

This is especially true for procedures involving use of a fiber-optic scope. More and more procedures may be performed these days through a very small opening, with instruments that are guided by these tiny viewing scopes. Surgeons need to have trained intensively to use these precision instruments well. If you've chosen an older surgeon but your procedure may be performed with these relatively new instruments, you shouldn't focus on how long the surgeon has been operating on your particular problem (he may well have been doing that for decades); the more pertinent question is, how long has he been doing it with the scope and through a minimal incision?

If the answer is in months, not years, or in fewer than dozens of procedures, you might want to rethink the match between the surgeon and the procedure. You might opt instead to have the same older surgeon do your operation, but with a conventional full-size incision—the way he's most comfortable operating.

**In some cases, younger can actually mean more experienced.**
If you are set on having your procedure performed using any techniques or instruments that have been introduced only in the last several years, you will probably be better served by a younger surgeon than an "old hand." Younger surgeons may have completed all their training using the current higher-tech methods, and so, paradoxically, are actually more experienced and proficient than others who may have decades on them in simple calendar terms.

**Your gut feeling counts. If the surgeon doesn't leave you feeling you're not just in good hands, but in *great* hands, keep looking.**
I think this recommendation speaks for itself.

**Get a second opinion.**
Your insurance company may require this. If not, it's still an excellent idea. It gives you the opportunity to talk to an independent medical evaluator, someone who has no vested interest in getting your business.

Find the second opinion much as you did the first—by asking other doctors, doing research to find out who the experts are, and asking friends and family members for names of doctors to call.

Don't ask your surgeon to recommend the second opinion; you risk the very real possibility that you will only get the name of a like-thinking doctor. It's not that your first choice is trying to skew the odds his way; it's just that it's normal for doctors to hold in high regard those who take a similar medical approach to cases.

## Beware of any doctor who discourages you from getting a second opinion.

It's fine to tell your doctor that you're seeking a second opinion. Good doctors don't feel threatened by the thought that others are reviewing their cases. However, if your doctor does object, or tells you not to go to anyone else, take that as a warning sign: It could be that his treatment plan doesn't conform to medical standards. The boxed text below tells what can happen when patients see a doctor who won't allow others to review his work.

---

*Here's a chilling story* from the headlines of the 1990s that is still useful as a cautionary tale for any patient who doubts the value of an independent second opinion. Dr. Cecil Jacobson was a fertility specialist with a booming practice in the northern Virginia suburbs of Washington, D.C. He told many of his patients that he had developed a new method of boosting a woman's chance to conceive. It involved injecting patients with the hormone hCG over a number of consecutive days.

After the patient had finished the series of shots, she was told to come in to take a pregnancy test. The test he administered works by detecting the level of hCG in the patient's urine, but Dr. Jacobson had been artificially raising the level with the shots, which meant that the pregnancy test would always come out positive. A few weeks past the time of the supposed "positive" pregnancy test, he would perform a sonogram. While the patient looked at the dark and grainy images on the screen, Dr. Jacobson would point out what he said were the outlines of the fetal head or identify a light streak as a developing spinal cord. But when, a week or two later, the patient would get her period and call the doctor to report that fact, he would tell her that she must have miscarried. He would then urge her to come back for another series of treatments, and the whole process would begin again. Many of his patients came back month after month. One patient was fooled into thinking she had been pregnant but miscarried *eight times*. When some patients openly wondered

---

whether they should seek a second opinion, Dr. Jacobson warned them not to. Other doctors, he explained, did not understand his "revolutionary" methods. If they wanted to have babies, they should just trust him, he said, and let him take care of them as he knew best.

But eventually some patients did consult other doctors, only to be told that, in all likelihood, they had never been pregnant. One of those patients tipped off a local Washington TV station, WRC, which sent an investigative reporter to check out the doctor's practice. She went through the series of hCG shots and then was asked to turn in a urine test, but instead of giving her own urine, she brought in a sample produced by a male colleague at the TV news department. It didn't matter—Dr. Jacobson still told her she was pregnant!

Once they saw their doctor exposed on a TV news show as a fraud, other patients quickly realized what he'd been doing to them, and the malpractice suits started pouring in. Dr. Jacobson had to close his practice. Not long afterward, he was defending himself against criminal charges as well—as it turned out, unsuccessfully. The doctor ended up losing his license and serving a sentence of five years in a federal penitentiary.

This denouement might have arrived years earlier if only a few of his patients had been quicker to seek an outside opinion of Dr. Jacobson's work.

**Educate yourself fully about your procedure and its aftermath.**
Before you go ahead and schedule your surgery, you ought to know as much as you can about how it's supposed to solve (or at least alleviate) your medical problem and how it's typically performed. Having such knowledge in advance will help you in your first meeting with the surgeon to understand what he or she is telling you. It will also help you to know what information your doctor needs from you. Perhaps most important, it will help you to notice if your surgeon

says anything that seems to be greatly at variance with what you've read. Your goal in educating yourself is not to make yourself into an expert, it's to be able to ask intelligent questions and have some basis from which to evaluate the answers.

By educating yourself about your procedure, you will also be prepared in the event that your surgeon (whom you picked by reputation of being the best in your area at doing the procedure you need) turns out not to be the best at communicating with patients. Unfortunately, many doctors speak only in jargon or don't give enough time to answer patients' questions fully—and quite frequently, patients don't even know what questions to ask. This can lead to last-minute confrontations and accusations, for example: "But doctor—no one told me I'd be unable to drive for six weeks afterward! Now I'll have to pull my kids out of day camp because I have no other way to get them there!" Or "What do you mean, I might need blood during the procedure? If I'd known that, I would have arranged to donate my own blood in advance."

You should have no trouble finding the information you seek. Each of the boldfaced headings below describes one way of increasing your knowledge. You may want to try some or all of the suggestions.

**Read books.**

In the publishing world today the "health and wellness" category is right up there with diet and cooking as one of the biggest, broadest, and most popular categories of nonfiction. Just go to any large bookstore and you'll find shelf after shelf devoted to medical problems, broken down by subtopic, with at least one, and quite possibly dozens, of titles for any disease, disorder, or condition you can name. Cancer, heart disease, women's health issues, chronic pain, and arthritis are some examples of subjects for which you can find more than a hundred books in print each.

To get a sense of how easy it is to find books on a specific medical problem, I asked my research assistant to visit to the Amazon.com website and look under the search term "cancer." Within a few clicks she found 474 books. They were grouped under ten subtopics: bone cancer, brain cancer, breast cancer, childhood leukemia, colorectal cancer, leukemia, lung cancer, lymphatic cancer, prostate cancer, and skin cancer. At random she chose "colorectal" and in an instant saw that there were forty-five titles available, including one by a doctor written under the aegis of the American Cancer Society, several books by patients, a few books focused on prevention, a couple that were compilations of articles on different issues within the subtopic, and finally, a few apiece about a specific type of surgery or treatment regimen for colon or rectal cancer. For each book carried by Amazon it was possible to read both professional reviewers' comments and reviews written by general readers.

While you probably want to be able to browse through the available books in real life, it helps to have a sense of what's in print before you go to the library or bookstore. As you browse, stop and read a paragraph or two at random, to be sure that the book you buy is written in clear, non-technical language that you can follow without needing a medical dictionary. Check out the writer's credentials: Is the book by a board certified M.D.? Someone who's performed the major procedures in the field for many years? Some of most helpful books have a foreword by a doctor but are written by former patients. These aren't strictly speaking medical books, but they can give you a very thorough sense of what it will be like to experience certain treatment regimens; the author has already done what you're about to go through and has survived to tell you what he or she has learned from the process.

Keep in mind that you don't have to buy books to read them. Any well stocked library should carry health care books written for a general audience. In addition, the librarian will be able to help you more quickly find those books describing the sort of procedure you are set to undergo.

### Use the Internet.

A vast, though unwieldy, source of information is the Internet, but as most experienced cyber-surfers have learned, it's often a challenge to tell the useful information from the nonsensical. There are websites, chat rooms, newsgroups, and bulletin boards for every imaginable disease or condition; some are by reputable doctors, nurses, or other health professionals; others are by quacks and imposters masquerading as experts.

Many of the more useful medical websites I've found are listed in Appendix D of this book.

### A good starting point for finding reading material about your condition is your own doctor.

Before Maryann had her last knee surgery, she had stumbled across information on the Internet about an innovative substance called "bone putty." It was designed to repair the kind of small holes that bone screws leave behind after they are removed. During her pre-operative appointment, in which she and her surgeon discussed the need to remove an old bone screw, Maryann asked if her surgeon was familiar with bone putty. Without hesitation, the doctor reached into a file and pulled out a copy of the journal literature on it. Not only did Maryann have reliable information, but her confidence in the surgeon also soared.

### One important caution: Take any advice from laypersons with a healthy dose of skepticism.

What works for one person in one set of circumstances is no guarantee it will work for you—and it could well be dangerous, to boot. Besides, you may have no way to find out whether the person pushing a particular procedure or cure is truthful and accurate in his or her account. All kinds of people with all kinds of motives use the Internet to push their personal agendas. Some are shilling for makers of certain supplements or devices. Others may be ranting about this or that procedure because they hold a grudge against some individual involved in their care who performed it on them. You just can't be sure.

So to be safe, you and your doctor should always discuss in detail any Internet-origin treatments or ideas about your health care needs, and you should always make sure you have your doctor's explicit approval before you act on any advice you may have received from someone in cyberspace.

### Visit QuackWatch.com.

One good way to protect yourself against worthless or harmful treatments and discredited techniques is to check the warnings on *www.quackwatch.com*. You can navigate the site by any number of ways, including searching by the name of the procedure or treatment you wish to check out, searching by category, or going to the site's index to see what's listed. Quackwatch.com not only provides papers and articles written by doctors or scientists debunking unproven or harmful "cures," but it also provides a forum for debate about medical controversies. If you're considering a procedure that is not wholly accepted by the mainstream medical community, you can read about it, pro and con, then bring any questions and concerns to your doctor, and put all the information together to make a rational decision on whether the procedure is right for you.

**Talk to others who have had the same condition/treatment.**
Earlier in this chapter I suggested that you ask around to find out if anyone you know can recommend a surgeon from personal experience. When you find someone who's already experienced what you're about to go through, you should do a lot more than just ask for a name: Pick that person's brain. Ask what they know now about the condition and its treatment that they wish they'd known right from the start. Keep in mind, however, that some people like to keep their medical details private. You must ask politely, and if the person declines, respect that desire for privacy. Fortunately, I think you'll discover that most former patients want to be helpful. They want to help others avoid pain and distress. They may also be able to recommend books or other sources of information that they found helpful, themselves. But as with information gleaned from strangers over the Internet, you should still keep the layperson's advice in perspective, remembering that each individual's case is unique and that your medical problem and its treatment might require a different course of action.

Again, always check with your doctor before putting anyone's lay advice into practice.

**Join a support group or association of patients with your condition.**
There are too many such groups to list here. But let me give you a real-life example that shows how useful these patient-driven organizations can be:

A husband and wife, both good friends of mine, had been trying to have a baby for years without luck. The wife was advised to have several invasive tests performed: a hysterosalpingogram, an endometrial biopsy, and a diagnostic laparoscopy. The last test needed to be performed in the hospital under general anesthesia. They wondered, What are all these tests for? Are they all really necessary? Are they part of the standard infertility work-up? Did they have to be done in any particular order?

This wasn't at all my area of expertise, so I couldn't advise them, but then they learned about RESOLVE, a national infertility support group and information clearinghouse. They visited that organization's website and found that there were pamphlets available on each procedure they were set to undergo. There were lay staff members available to answer questions or refer questions to qualified medical experts. They joined the organization, and even now, years later, after they successfully conceived and had two children as the result of medical intervention, they still are members of RESOLVE, to continue to help others.

To find a support group that fits your own situation, try using a reliable Internet search engine, like Google.com, Ask.com, or About.com. Go to the "search" box and type in the name of your disease or condition and "association" or "organization."

My research associate tested this out by seeing if she could find an association or support group for a friend suffering from a gynecological condition known as endometriosis. The friend had been advised to have a hysterectomy to relieve the constant pain of the disease. My assistant went to Ask.com, which allows questions to be typed in normal English, and typed: "Is there an association for endometriosis patients?" The very first website that popped up in response was that of the Endometriosis Association, which describes itself this way:

> The Endometriosis Association (EA) is a non-profit, self-help organization founded by women for women. The EA is dedicated to providing information and support to women and girls with endometriosis, educating the public as well

as the medical community about the disease, and conducting and promoting research related to endometriosis.

That was exactly what this woman was looking for. After contacting the organization, she was quickly put in touch with other patients who had had a hysterectomy or other treatments, and they helped her decide whether the recommended surgical solution was right for her.

## Understand your non-surgical alternatives and why they may or may not be suitable in your case.

Nobody wants to undergo unnecessary surgeries. If there are alternatives that yield the same or better results for patients like you, you should know about them. Surgeons naturally tend to be biased in favor of quick surgical solutions. Other doctors may take a more conservative approach. In the section above, I cited the case of a woman with endometriosis whose doctor had advised her to have a hysterectomy. See the boxed story below to find out how she explored her non-surgical alternatives and what the outcome was.

*Hannah was a married woman* in her mid-thirties who, almost from her first menstrual period at age thirteen, had experienced pain and excessive bleeding. The older she got, the worse her condition became. The diagnosis was endometriosis.

Hannah learned as much as she could about the disease, borrowing books from the library and meeting and corresponding with former endometriosis patients. One thing quickly became clear: Endometriosis is not well understood; there are various theories about what causes it and many different treatment options, and all of them are to one degree or another controversial. Some doctors take a conservative approach, recommending trial and error over time to see if hormones or other medications work to suppress or reverse its symptoms. Others say the condition isn't actually a disease at all, and that endometriosis appears in one degree or another in most women; such doctors tend to adopt a "wait and see" attitude, leaving the symptoms untreated except in the most extreme cases. However, many gynecological surgeons insist that the best thing to do is go into the woman's pelvis and laser away all the endometriosis adhesions that can be found. Still, endometriosis tends to return, and once a woman experiences the return of symptoms after laser treatment, she might consider hysterectomy as a permanent solution.

Hannah pondered her options. As she explained, "Endometriosis is a disease of decisions; there is no right answer." At first she decided to give drug therapy a try, but she quickly concluded it wasn't effective in her severe case. Then she tried the laser treatment, but the adhesions returned within a few months. By that time she had done quite a lot of research and even more thinking about how the various different treatment options suited her own sense of her health-care needs. She had already had a child, and although she would have liked to have had another, she knew that her fertility was already severely curtailed by the progress of the disease. She had found at best only temporary relief from the more conservative measures she had tried, and she was ready to put the disease behind her—even if it meant the end of her dream of having more children. So Hannah went back to the gynecological surgeon who had advised her to have the hysterectomy and set a date for the procedure. Now, many years later—years that have been pain free—she is sure that she made the right decision.

# CHAPTER 2

# Choosing the Best Hospital for Safety and Comfort

Finding a good hospital isn't like finding a good inn or resort, but wouldn't it be nice if it were? You could ask friends to recommend someplace nice to go. You could read reviews looking for that one place that seems best suited to your particular occasion to visit (and imagine the sort of thing a reviewer would say: "Mercy General … perfect for that intimate little mid-week break to part with your old gall bladder")! You could focus on things you really understand and appreciate, like the taste of the food and the feel of the bed linens, and the friendliness and efficiency of the staff. But unfortunately for most patients, the choice involves far more than the physical comforts of the place. You'll need to find out how often the particular procedure you'll be having is performed at various hospitals and what kinds of outcomes each hospital has. You'll want to know about the availability of advanced equipment and new treatment techniques (and you'll probably have to learn a lot of new terms, even to ask the right questions). You'll be concerned with what other medical experts have to say about the hospital—and much, much more.

Getting the answers to these kinds of questions may seem a daunting task. It needn't be, if you approach it step by step, starting with this tip:

## Let your surgeon guide your choice of hospitals.

Once you have found a surgeon you like and trust, you have found your best advisor about the place to have the procedure performed.

Your surgeon will tell you to which hospitals he or she is allowed to admit patients.

Many surgeons have privileges at more than one, which means that you can choose among them, based on your own evaluation of the pros and cons. You will consider many, many factors, both practical and medical, as you make your choice, among them: hospital reputation; availability of the services you need; location; parking; visiting hours and other visitor policy matters (such as, "Are there limits on how many visitors?"); room size and availability of private rooms; food; religious affiliation; and many others considered in this chapter.

One of the biggest factors—and for all but the richest patients, the most limiting—in your choice is the sort of health insurance you have. Always check with your insurance company before scheduling any surgery. (More on this point in Chapter 5, "Taking Care of Business.")

Not all the factors influencing your hospital choice are equal. Questions involving your comfort and convenience are important, of course, but unless your surgery is the most routine sort, done with minimal anesthesia, you'll want to assign the highest priority to finding the hospital with the best track record for good outcomes in the medical procedure you will be undergoing.

Don't assume that your surgeon will be collecting such statistics for you. In most cases, it will be up to you to weigh the pros and cons of the different hospitals yourself and make a choice. The sections that follow suggest ways to find the information you seek.

## Check accreditation.

Since 1951, the *Joint Commission on Accreditation of Healthcare Organizations* has worked through its system of accreditation to improve the safety and quality of care provided to the public. The JCAHO evaluates and accredits more than 19,500 health care organizations in the United States, including hospitals, health care networks, managed care organizations, and health care organizations that provide home care, long-term care, behavioral health care, laboratory, and ambulatory care services. A not-for-profit group, the JCAHO is considered the world's leading health care standards-setting and accrediting body. To conduct the accreditation survey, the JCAHO employs more than

650 physicians, nurses, health-care administrators, medical technologists, psychologists, respiratory therapists, pharmacists, durable medical equipment providers, and social workers.

During a JCAHO audit, a survey team of the board considers safety practices, adherence to Occupational Safety and Health Administration (OSHA) standards, record keeping, drug control procedures, patient rights, and many other areas. To earn and maintain accreditation, an organization must undergo an on-site survey at least every three years. Laboratories must be surveyed every two years.

Organizations can get a passing grade, or a passing grade with commendation; they can also be put on probation, or even shut down. The JCAHO provides a comprehensive guide on the Internet to help individuals learn more about the quality of health-care organizations. Go to www.jcaho.org and click on the link to Quality Check™ to see the list of the JCAHO-accredited health-care organizations and programs in the United States. The Quality Check listing includes each organization's name, address, telephone number, accreditation decision, accreditation date, and current accreditation status and effective date.

You can also check the individual performance reports for many accredited health organizations. Performance reports provide more detailed information about an organization's operations, including comparisons with similar organizations. Copies of certain reports aren't available on-line, but you can get them by calling the JCAHO's Customer Service Center at 630-792-5800.

**To be sure the hospital's rating is up to date, find out when it went through its last accreditation review.**

In a spring 1999, four-part series in the *Boston Globe* on hospital errors, reporter Larry Tye described the intense preparation undertaken by Westerly (Rhode Island) Hospital before the visit by JCAHO inspectors: "Westerly staffers really might have been scared if they weren't so thoroughly prepared. They'd been rehearsing for a year, with nearly 30 drills on everything from how to keep track of drugs to when to keep patients restrained." When you know the inspection was recent—or is scheduled for the near future, you can figure that everyone in the hospital has been brushing up on their skills and paying special attention to safety procedures.

**Check with any hospital watchdog organizations in your area.**
Your state or region should have a public or nonprofit watchdog organization that publishes failure-rate information about hospitals. If you're not sure, call your state or local government citizen information line, or call your local Chamber of Commerce and ask for information about either government or private organizations that maintain track records on hospital performance.

For example, in Cleveland, Ohio, hospitals are required to publish their failure rates for certain procedures. In Massachusetts, both the Department of Public Health and the private Massachusetts Coalition for the Prevention of Medical Errors are involved in record-keeping of medical errors. With a few telephone calls—or possibly with some surfing through cyberspace—you should be able to find out who compiles such information in your own state.

A particularly useful website for patients, no matter which state they live in, is the one maintained by the Public Citizen Health Research Group at *www.citizen.org/hrg/*, which, among other things, posts notices of "confirmed violations, civil infractions and narratives of selected case reports" from 527 hospitals that it rates among the nation's worst.

**Check *US News & World Report's* "Hospital Ratings" issue.**
This special issue of the weekly news magazine is published once a year, usually in July. The various regional editions of the magazine include a "Best in Your Area" feature. But you don't need to wait for the newsstand issue to appear; you can check the magazine's website to see the rankings at any time of year by going to: *www.usnews.com/usnews/nycu/health/hosptl/tophosp.htm*.

Hospitals are ranked for each of the major specialties (cancer, digestive disorders, otolaryngology, geriatrics, gynecology, heart, hormonal disorders, kidney/nephrology, neurology and neurosurgery, orthopedics, respiratory disorders, rheumatology, and urology, plus shorter, less detailed listings on hospital treatment of eye disease, psychiatry, pediatrics, and rehabilitation). The magazine explains the fourteen factors that go into compiling a hospital's score; among these are: "reputational score," that is, the percentage of physicians who identified the hospital in response to the _US News & World Report_ survey question; mortality ratio, a comparison of the actual to expected deaths of Medicare patients from admission through discharge in a three-year period; technology services, a list of key technological services that the most advanced hospitals are expected to provide; and ratio of registered nurses to beds.

Because of the comprehensiveness of its survey and the sound methods used to create the index and rankings, the _US News & World Report_ rankings are generally taken by the medical community to be a dependable guide for patients to use in making their hospital choice.

## Understand your choices of different types of hospitals.

There's more to hospital choice that finding out which has the best success rate for this or that procedure. You also have personal, religious, family, and employment considerations. Let's say you're having routine hernia surgery. You don't need an ultra-high-tech center. Once you've chosen a surgeon you trust, who has got a good track record, you probably don't have to worry too much about the hospital's ranking on a national level. Just be sure you're choosing only from among accredited places and that there are no ongoing scandals.

Once you've done that, you can start looking at the other non-medical issues that play a role in your comfort and emotional health. For example, will you be able to be visited by your children during the day? Will the food conform to your religious requirements? Is the hospital close to your home?

To answer these questions you have to know something about the different types of hospitals and the advantages and disadvantages of each:

There are **general hospitals,** which are usually located in a large urban or regional center and are able to provide the broadest range of services.

There are **community hospitals,** which tend to be smaller, lacking the most advanced care. They may not be part of a university program, so there are no medical students to bother you, but also no teaching doctors in attendance there—and teaching doctors tend to be the tops in their field. Eager and thorough medical students tend to pore over the details of their patients' cases, looking to learn something new and interesting, which older doctors seldom do.

There are **teaching hospitals,** which do assign medical students to cases—and while the students won't have the sure, skilled touch of a long-experienced doctor or nurse, they will have boundless enthusiasm and curiosity and may study your case with an interest in the details that the older personnel no longer have.

There are **specialized hospitals** that only work with a certain type of patient; for example: pediatric hospitals that just treat children; veterans hospitals just for former members of the military; maternity hospitals that are only for pregnant women; or women's hospitals that deal with the full range of women's health problems. There are also orthopedic hospitals, coronary care hospitals, cancer treatment centers, rehabilitation hospitals, long-term care facilities, and an array of others grouped by specialty, either in freestanding facilities or as a separate building of a larger hospital center.

There are **hospitals affiliated with religious organizations,** which can provide clergy members to visit and comfort you and help you observe the rituals of your faith during your stay. But there may be restrictions on medical procedures that conflict with the teachings of that faith: For example, a Catholic hospital will not perform an abortion, except to save the life of the mother. Religiously affiliated hospitals may have their own rules that supersede a patient's "do not resuscitate" order. You may be required to undergo heroic measures to keep you alive. (For more discussion about this issue, see the sections on Advance Health Care Directives in Chapter 5, "Taking Care of Business.")

Keep in mind that these categories often overlap. Take for example, Georgetown University Hospital in Washington, DC. It belongs in four different categories: It's a large, general hospital serving the greater Washington metropolitan area. It contains within it a specialized hospital, the Vincent Lombardi Cancer Center. It's a teaching hospital with faculty and students from the Georgetown

University Medical School. And it's religiously affiliated with the Roman Catholic Church.

The table on page 34 lists the hospital types I've mentioned and outlines some of the advantages and disadvantages of each. Of course,

---

**Here's how Marsha Wise** went about her search for a rehabilitation facility for her husband, David, who had suffered a cerebral hemorrhage, brain surgery, and a massive stroke. First, she investigated two nationally known facilities in her area, along with a community hospital that had converted one floor into a rehabilitation unit.

Here's what she was seeking:

- Intensity of the therapy program
- Responsiveness of staff
- Caring atmosphere
- Proximity to their home (since she would need to come and go frequently).

After due consideration of all the pros and cons, she chose the community hospital's rehab center.

Marsha didn't just make the best choice for her husband; she also took what she'd learned from her hospital search experience and translated it into a form that others could use—a brochure with tips for choosing the right rehabilitation facilities. To get a copy, send a stamped, self-addressed envelope to:

TIPS
PO Box 596
Middletown, MD 21769

Donations to defray printing costs are accepted but not required. For information about ordering quantities, email tips@xecu.net (with "rehab" in the subject line).

---

| Hospital Type | Typical Advantages | Typical Disadvantages |
|---|---|---|
| **General hospital** | Provides a broad range of services<br><br>Serves greater metropolitan area or region and so can attract top names in each field | May be very large and impersonal |
| **Community hospital** | Less likely to employ novices just completing their education<br><br>Less likelihood of disruptions of rest because of rounds, questions from staff in training, etc.<br><br>Flexibility in care and procedures (for example, in visiting hours) | May be small and lacking specialists on staff<br><br>May lack high-tech equipment or resources to diagnose and treat complex problems |
| **Specialized hospital** | Expertise and resources to provide superior care in a particular area of medicine or with a particular category of patient (for example, children)<br><br>Presence of specialists and subspecialists of many kinds | Limited ability to diagnose and treat a broad range of problems (for example, the orthopedic patient who develops a coronary problem)<br><br>Limited ability to provide care for patients who fall outside the category of patient treated (for example, the baby born at a maternity hospital who needs neonatal intensive care and has to be transferred to a pediatric hospital) |
| **Teaching hospital** | Intellectual curiosity of new professionals comes into play in diagnosis and treatment<br><br>Collegial atmosphere encourages exchange of ideas<br><br>Availability of (or at least awareness of) experimental and cutting-edge therapies | Number of novices present can be disruptive and confusing to the patients<br><br>Participation of novices in patient care can expose patients to unnecessary pain or inconvenience |
| **Religiously affiliated hospital** | Provides pastoral care to patients who wish it<br><br>Is concerned with non-medical aspects of care; integrates patient's beliefs and values into care | May refuse to perform certain procedures that conflict with religious doctrine (for example, Catholic hospitals do not perform abortions or provide advanced fertility treatments)<br><br>May have own rules for end-of-life care that conflict with patient's own wishes not to have "heroic measures" taken to preserve life |

this list is far from comprehensive. It's just intended to give you an overview of the main hospital types. To get specific answers about any particular hospital, see the following tip about taking a hospital tour.

## Go on a hospital tour.

This is a routine thing for pregnant women to do when choosing a hospital for labor and delivery, but you may not have known it was an option for other types of patients as well. It's rare that a hospital would turn down a request to tour their facilities—and I would be extremely wary of any hospital that did. Of course, to protect patients' privacy, you cannot go into any occupied rooms, but you certainly should expect to be shown an unoccupied room, the nurses' station, the cafeteria, the lounge, various waiting rooms, and other public areas. To schedule your tour, call the public relations department of the hospital of interest to you, or call the general information line and ask for your call to be routed to the right department.

When taking your tour, bring along a small notebook and take notes. Pay attention to cleanliness, noise level, and level of activity (which may be busy—that's fine—but it should not seem frenzied or chaotic). Look around at the rooms that are open to your view and take note of any that seem particularly nice (or any you'd want to avoid); you might be able to get a requested room if the hospital isn't crowded during your stay. Ask questions about anything that strikes you as problematic. For example, if you see that one of the elevators is out of service, ask, how long it has been broken and when is it going to be fixed?

Your tour guide may not be able to answer all your questions on the spot, but if she's good at her job, she'll promise to follow up by calling or writing to you with whatever information she's been unable to supply during your visit.

A well-conducted hospital tour can do a lot more than help you decide on which hospital to choose. When you have the chance to familiarize yourself with the place where you'll be staying during your procedure and recovery, you can prepare yourself, in both practical and emotional terms, for the experience you can expect to have there.

## Don't judge a hospital by its name alone.

Don't assume, for example, that a hospital with "General" in its name can't provide specialized care. Many large general hospitals have specialized sub-units within them. Massachusetts General Hospital is an excellent example of a general hospital that is also a mecca for top specialists and a place where patients can find cutting-edge therapies.

Another mistake patients commonly make is to avoid religiously affiliated hospitals if they're not a member of that religious group. New York Presbyterian happens to be one of the finest hospitals in the country for all types of patients—definitely not just Presbyterians. There are Jewish hospitals, Catholic hospitals, Mormon hospitals, Baptist hospitals, Methodist hospitals, hospitals of almost every faith you can name, but all sharing a commitment to heal the sick, of whatever faith. You might lean toward going to a hospital affiliated with your own faith for the comfort you get from seeing familiar clergy in the halls, but let that be just one among many factors influencing your choice.

If you are in doubt as to what type of care a particular hospital can provide, don't speculate, but call the hospital's administrative or public relations office and get factual answers to your specific questions.

## Do choose a specialized hospital if you neatly fit the category of patient that the hospital was designed to treat.

There's no question in my mind that children, for example, are better off being treated in pediatric hospitals. When your child is in the pediatric wing of a general hospital, he may end up intubated with a tube that's too large, or the person starting his IV line may not have access to a "butterfly," the fine needle used in most pediatric hospitals for children's smaller veins.

If you have a bone problem, in most cases you'll be better off in an orthopedic hospital, so that you'll be assured that the aides who are lifting you into your shower seat are all trained about how to keep your limb elevated, rather than taking your chances at a general hospital, where the aides might have received some specialized training … or they might not have.

But see the following tip for advice about when *not* to choose a specialized hospital.

**If you have multiple problems affecting separate organs or systems, *don't* go to a specialized hospital.**

The main disadvantage to a specialized hospital is that its staff may be too focused on the particular set of problems it was designed to treat. Let's say you're going to an orthopedic hospital for knee surgery, but you've lately been feeling some shortness of breath, and occasionally, a painful tightness in your chest. You might not think much about it—and it's quite possible that your mild symptoms would not set off any alarm bells on your pre-admission tests—and so you go into the orthopedic hospital not realizing you have an incipient heart condition. Now suppose you have a heart attack while recovering from knee surgery. If you were in a large general hospital, there would be cardiac specialists on hand to give you immediate, advanced care. You'd be moved right away from the orthopedic wing to the cardiac wing. But at the specialized hospital it might take longer for staff to correctly diagnose what was happening to you; then a cardiac specialist would have to be brought in to treat you, or else you would have to be transferred to a different hospital.

The possibility of needing to switch hospitals should definitely be a consideration for the woman who chooses a maternity hospital for labor and delivery. If it happens that her baby is born with a severe problem—a stressful situation for any parent—there will be the added stress of seeing the newborn rushed by ambulance from the maternity hospital to a children's hospital, where the baby can receive the advanced neonatal intensive care required. In a large general hospital the neonatal intensive care unit will be close to the maternity unit, and pediatricians and maternal/fetal care specialists are used to working together closely.

**If you prefer to limit the number of strangers examining you, don't choose a teaching hospital (especially if your problem is straightforward and its treatment is simple to administer).**

In a teaching hospital you can expect to have students, interns, and residents involved in your case, as well as your own doctor and nurses and other caregivers. If your problem or its treatment is at all unusual, you may find yourself the object of constant attention.

This can be good or bad, depending on your situation and your personal inclination.

It can be good if your case is complicated and not responding well to the usual treatments, because a multiplicity of people concerned with your problem means a multiplicity of people who could come up with the particular solution you need. Interns and residents are usually bright, hardworking, and interested in having input whenever possible. When you have several earnest young med students discussing your case with each other and with their supervising physician, or researching articles and studies for information that could lead to a new treatment approach, you reap the benefits of the teaching hospital system.

But when your case is just another appendectomy, like many thousands that have come before it, and all you want to do is rest quietly and recover, you don't need some overeager twenty-three-year-old waking you to ask you the same questions that your own doctor asked you two hours earlier.

On the other hand, teaching hospitals tend to attract the best doctors and have the latest experimental equipment. Sometimes it's worth putting up with the presence of students and other learners in order to receive medical care from doctors so experienced and knowledgeable that they are qualified to teach others.

### Choose a community hospital when you value closeness and convenience—and your case doesn't call for cutting-edge technology.

Because a community hospital means just that—in your community—you won't have to travel far to get there. You'll probably find a large, low-cost parking lot, too. (With all the high costs associated with your hospital care, every little bit helps!) Unless the community hospital has ties to a university medical school, you won't have the disruptions common to a teaching hospital, you probably won't have novices drawing your blood, and your care is likely to be more flexible. I remember my father saying that when he began his practice, hospitalized patients who were alcoholics used to be given a glass of wine in the evening to ease their withdrawal symptoms—well, that's flexibility in the extreme. But even in this day and age I've heard of community hospitals where visiting hours are whatever the patients and nurses like and where patients can order pizzas from the neighborhood delivery service. So if you're having something done that you are assured can be handled safely and effectively just about everywhere, by all means, arrange to have it done where you can also get a delivery of your favorite, the Neapolitan Special with anchovies and extra garlic.

**For complicated surgery or surgery to deal with a life-threatening condition, choose a hospital that does a lot of that procedure; in other words, you _do_ want to be on an "assembly line."**

You probably won't find yourself shopping for a hospital unless you have a serious medical problem and have already consulted more than one physician. If that describes your situation, then you want to choose a hospital with teams of professionals used to working together, with years of experience helping patients with your disease, injury, or condition. When it comes to surgery, "practice makes perfect" is more than a tired cliché, it's a practical tip that should strongly influence your choice.

**Find out whether the hospital has the latest in drugs and equipment used to treat your specific condition and its complications or side effects.**

In the next two chapters, "The Pre-surgery Interview" and "All About Anesthesia," you will learn what questions and concerns you should raise with your surgeon and with your anesthesiologist if you fall into any of several categories (for example, if you have diabetes or asthma, or are a smoker). In some cases, I'll be suggesting specific therapies or treatment options to ask about, so you'll need to find out whether the hospital you've chosen is one that will allow you to make use of those options. Check those chapters for the names of the specific drugs or technologies to ask about when investigating your hospital choices.

**Find out what you can about any labor problems at the hospital.**

You don't want to have surgery on the day the nurses go out on strike—

or the maintenance staff or nurse's aides. If there are labor contract negotiations underway and a strike is threatened, your local newspapers should be on top of the situation. If you check the headlines of recent days' issues and see nothing on the subject, then for added assurance, you might try logging onto the newspaper's website and running a search for the terms "hospital" and "strike" to see if anything turns up.

You might think all you'd have to do is call the hospital and ask an administrative official if the labor situation is stable. I wouldn't bother—they might lie to you, or at least try to minimize any impending problems. Asking the nurses or aides directly is more likely to yield useful information—that is, if any trouble is actually brewing.

What if you're set on a certain hospital, because it meets your criteria for safety and convenience, but you learn that a strike is possible? I would strongly advise you to delay your surgery until the situation is resolved and the nurses are back on the job. A hospital may limp along with a skeleton crew, but the quality of patient care will certainly suffer as a result.

If the procedure cannot be put off, then search for a hospital unaffected by the labor problem.

## Find out about any plans for the hospital's physical plant.

Imagine this scenario: You've just had treatment for a collapsed lung. Breathing is still painful, and you feel exhausted all the time. All you want to do is rest. But construction workers are renovating the floor you're on. There's construction dust swirling around and electric tools are relentlessly banging, drilling, and sawing. What a nightmare!

And you could have avoided it by having thought to ask a few simple questions before your scheduled your procedure. "Tell me about any renovation plans that the hospital has." Ask about the specific ward or wing where patients in your category usually stay.

It's fine for hospitals to upgrade and improve their facilities—it's just that you don't want to be there while they do. Of course, scheduling so as to be housed in the completed renovated part is great, if you can arrange it.

**If you find that local choices can't fully meet your needs, consider traveling to a hospital with a nationwide or global reputation.**

Some hospitals attract patients from all over the world—for good reason. For some of these patients, these faraway hospitals offer the best—perhaps the only—hope of survival. John Hopkins University Hospital in Baltimore, Maryland, has run programs for AIDS patients using experimental drugs not available anywhere else. The Cleveland Clinic in Cleveland, Ohio, has pioneered several new procedures in open-heart surgery. The Mayo Clinic in Rochester, Minnesota, is top rated in so many specialties and sub-specialties, it's impossible to single out any one department.

If you have thoroughly investigated the medical services available in your own region and find that you need experimental or innovative techniques that you can only get far from home, then pack and prepare yourself for a trip.

The doctors who have so far been unable to provide the level of care you need close to home should be willing to assist you in making arrangements to be seen and treated elsewhere. Be sure to have copies of all relevant medical records sent so that tests won't have to be repeated and too much time won't be wasted.

# CHAPTER 3

# The Pre-surgery Interview: What Every Patient Needs to Know

After you have decided on a surgeon but before you actually go to the hospital for whatever you need to have done, you will have an office visit with your surgeon—perhaps several. At some point during your meeting you will almost certainly be asked to do either of two things (and many surgeons will have you do both):

- Have a long face-to-face interview in which you are asked a great many questions about your current state of health and your health history, including your family's health history.
- Fill out an extensive questionnaire about your current state of health and your own and your family's health history.

The tips that follow are intended to help you understand what information is important for your surgeon to know and how such information is used to make your hospital experience both safer and more comfortable for you.

As you read through the tips, you will undoubtedly find many that do not apply to your situation—just ignore those. But be sure to note all those that *do* apply to you, and if the suggestion is to ask your surgeon about a particular issue or do some digging into your family history to find out the answer to this or that question on the surgeon's questionnaire, make every effort to do so. None of the issues raised in this chapter is trivial, and quite a few could make the difference between a short, uneventful hospital stay and one spent coping with all kinds of unfortunate consequences.

## Don't leave blanks on your pre-surgery questionnaire or health history form.

If you don't know how to answer a question or you don't understand what information is being sought, ask for clarification. Many patients fail to provide all the information the surgeon needs because they can't figure out what a question means. There is nothing wrong with asking, for example, "When it says 'List all past operations,' does dental surgery count? I had my wisdom teeth out under a local anesthetic plus nitrous oxide when I was nineteen."

*Don't worry about asking a stupid question.* If there's something that's not clear, then asking a question is really the smartest thing you can do. Even if you're fairly sure what information the question calls for, there's never any harm in double-checking. If the questionnaire uses any medical terminology unfamiliar to you, by all means get a definition. You're the patient; you didn't go to medical school, and there's no reason why you can't have things explained in layman's terms. It's the doctor's job or the office assistant's job to guide you through this often intimidating process—though you may have to prod them a little to get them to do their jobs properly. You are paying for this service, after all, so don't be shy about speaking up—especially since the success of your procedure could hinge upon the doctor having the right information ahead of time.

## Have the facts of your medical history available as you fill out your questionnaire.

Since you now know you are going to be asked to provide a detailed history, either orally or in writing or both, it makes sense to gather as much information on your medical background as you can ahead of time. Not many of us walk around with all the details of our own past medical problems stuffed in our memories. Yet small details in your history can in certain cases lead to big differences in your treatment. To be able to supply dates of past surgeries and dosages of medications taken long ago, it helps to have access to sources of information, as well as the time to do some research.

So it's best if your doctor can let you take home the questionnaire and then return it in a few days. That way you'll be able to call your mother across the country and ask if she remembers how old you were when you had meningitis; or you can look back over your old car insurance files to get the date of that accident in which you broke your leg and had it put back together with surgical pins.

## Get the details of your family's medical history straight so that your doctor can put your own health history in a larger context.

This means you may have to call relatives and ask, "Did Grandpa die of a heart attack or a stroke? About how old was he when it happened?"

Some patients resent all the personal information sought on health questionnaires. It's important to remember that medical information is completely confidential; doctors and nurses have no interest in your tangled family relationships, except those specific facts that are relevant to your medical diagnosis, treatment plan, and prognosis.

Let's take a difficult case as an example. A patient, John, knows that the person he grew up calling "Dad" is not his biological father. He knows it's a deep, dark family secret that his mother became pregnant with him during an affair but allowed her husband to believe himself to be the father. John is now struggling to fill out a health questionnaire with questions about his father's race, nationality, and history of certain genetic disorders. John should not put down anything about his legal father—that's not relevant to his own genetic history—nor should he attempt to explain on the form why his mother and his biological father were not married (the doctor doesn't need to know those particular intimate details). He simply needs to know some facts about the man whose genetic heritage is part of what makes John who he is now. If John doesn't know the answers, then he should do his best to find out what he can. If that means he must call his mother and ask her to help him complete his health questionnaire accurately, then he should put his embarrassment aside and do so. The outcome of his surgery could actually depend on it.

## Be completely frank about your own lifestyle.

When it comes to your health history, it's not just a question of accuracy about when you had chickenpox or whether or not you have a penicillin allergy; there's also the matter of your own conscious behavior that can affect your health. Too many patients are worried about keeping up appearances with the doctor, when what they ought to be worried about goes a lot deeper than their image. They know their doctor has told them to stop smoking and to drink no more than a glass or two of wine a day; yet they're still hooked on that pack-and-a-half a day and have been known to put away a more than a few bottles of beer in one sitting. They don't always know *why* they should admit that they're still smoking and drinking too much; they think there's no harm in fudging the facts "just a little bit."

Perhaps more to the point, many patients worry more about the doctor's reaction if they own up to their continuing bad habits. They think they'll get scolded, like naughty children, if they're found out. I wish that were the only consequence. But the fact is that alcohol can interfere with administration of anesthesia, and certain alcohol-anesthesia combinations can even be deadly. And when a surgeon knows his patient is a current smoker, he expects to find the circulatory and respiratory systems impaired to a certain degree and is prepared to deal with the problems he finds.

Getting wrong information will often lead the doctor to a wrong conclusion about the origins of a problem, and consequently a wrong approach to treatment. Candor in the pre-surgical interview should therefore be viewed as a simple form of preventive medicine.

### Be sure to report any drug allergies or adverse reactions to drugs.

Have you ever had a bad reaction to an antibiotic? Or an anesthetic, a narcotic, or any other type of drug (including over-the-counter ones)? Or have you been told that you once had a bad reaction to a drug when you were a small child? Report any such incidents with any and all detail you can provide: name of the drug, date or best guess as to the date (labeled as such), description of the reaction, how it was treated, name of the doctor who was treating you at the time. Don't worry about reporting incidents that may turn out to be irrelevant. It's far better to let the doctor spend some time assessing your potential to react to this or that drug *before* you go to the hospital than to skip over the issue and leave your surgical team to figure out how to cope with your swollen airway caused by an allergic reaction to a drug you should never have been given.

## Know the difference between an allergy and a sensitivity—but report your sensitivities, too.

An allergy is not the same as a sensitivity. When you're allergic to something, it means you are prone to get an *anaphylactic reaction,* that is, a series of events from a release of chemicals in your body that have

---

*Louise is sensitive to Demerol.* Here's her story:

When I had knee surgery at a hospital in Washington, DC, a nurse woke me up in the middle of the night with a shot in my leg. In seconds, I vomited all over her. "Is that Demerol?" I asked.

She seemed more interested in cleaning the vomit off her clothes than in answering my question. "Yes," she said. She seemed totally annoyed with me—as if this was my fault!

"Doesn't my chart indicate that I can't take Demerol?" I argued. I was in pain—how dare she get mad at me for her own mistake!

The room was dark. There was just the light from the hallway coming into my room. I saw the nurse take a quick look at the chart. Then she said, with an edge in her voice, "If you can't take Demerol, then all I can give you is Tylenol."

"Fine," I said.

"But I can't give it to you now because I've just given you the Demerol." Then she left the room!

The next morning, I told the head nurse and my doctor what had happened. I don't know if they took any action to improve that nurse's bedside manner or chart-reading skills, but I do know I didn't see her the next night.

---

dramatic results. Your throat will swell. You might get hives. Your circulation is affected. That is not the same as having a sensitivity to (for example) codeine that causes nausea. The story in the box on page 47 gives an example illustrating the importance of making your hospital care team aware of any drug sensitivities *before* you check into the hospital—and making sure you remind them again, before anything is put into your body.

**If you are currently taking any drugs, note on your pre-surgical questionnaire exactly what you're taking, how long you've been on them, what they're for, and who prescribed them.**

You may do this in either of two ways:

1. Before you go to your appointment for your pre-surgical interview, assemble the drugs you take (including over-the-counter drugs, vitamins, minerals, and any other supplements) and note on a piece of paper the exact name, including the brand name if known, of what you take, the dosage (usually listed on the container in "mg" [milligrams] or "mcg" [micrograms], and the instructions you are following as you take them (for example, "take three times a days with meals" or "take on an empty stomach upon waking and at bedtime").

or

2. Bring in the containers and pill bottles of everything you take and let the doctor or doctor's office staff see exactly what you're on and help you fill out the questionnaire based on the actual medications, supplements, and other pills that you've brought in.

Do the former if you are on only one or two or three drugs and are clear on what they are, when and how you take them, and what each is for. Do the latter if you're not entirely clear what the name of a particular drug actually is (for example, you don't know if it's a generic drug or a brand-name drug) or you're not sure about the dosage or whether you've been taking it according to the instructions that came with it. (See the story in the box on page 49 about some common mistakes patients make about their medications.) If it turns out you haven't been taking a drug according to your doctor's instructions, do be sure that this fact is noted on your health history.

*I've learned it's always a good idea* to double-check when my patients report what medications they're on. Some patients don't know the correct names of the drugs they take every day. That definitely gets in the way of communicating with hospital staff members trying to help them. I once asked a lady if she took any medications and she said, "Yes. I take 'Skif.'" She saw the initials "SKF" for SmithKline and French—the name of the pharmaceutical company on the package of the drug she used—and mistakenly thought that was the name of the pill. It would have been very difficult for me to figure out that she was taking Tagamet and know how to protect her against common drug interactions if she hadn't had a sample with her.

Mispronunciations can create the same kind of confusion. More than once, I've had a heart patient tell me he takes "Dick Johnson" instead of "digoxin" *(di-jock'-sin)*, because that's probably what it sounded like when his doctor pronounced it.

The simplest way to avoid this kind of confusion is to keep a written list of all your medications—and keep it updated.

## Report anything out of the ordinary when it comes to your experience with medications, both now and in the past.

For example, you are not on any medications currently, but five years ago when you had an injury, you were put on the regular adult dose of a muscle relaxant, which made you so drowsy that you sometimes fell asleep at work. Your doctor discovered that to remain alert, you needed the child's dose instead. This sort of disclosure tells your current doctor how you might react if you were put on the same medication or one of a similar class of drugs.

Conversely, you might be resistant to certain medications, as indicated by your response in the past. Report any such unexpected reactions, whether or not they led to a change in the medication or dosage you were prescribed, and whether or not you think your current medical problem could involve a drug of that type. Leave it to your doctor and medical team to determine if your past experiences might be relevant to your current condition and its treatment.

Never assume that the way you responded to a drug was all "in your head," that is, a byproduct of your psychological state at the time. Research has confirmed that our responses to drugs are largely governed by our genes. As a result, scientists are on the fast track to developing tests to guide doctors in prescribing drugs and determining dosages tailored to individual patients. I am optimistic that doctors will soon know with much more specificity who should get which drugs, and how much they should get to increase drug effectiveness and minimize side effects.

Gene-related drug reactions fall into five basic categories, and in reading over them as I have summarized them below, you may find yourself thinking, "Ah ha! I knew there must be a reason why I react that way when I take X drug."

### Five Types of Genetically Determined Responses to Medication

1. **Impact level:** Your genes play a role in determining how effective certain medications may be. For example, a person may have genes that cause a particular blood pressure medication to have a strong impact, while a person lacking those genes may find the same drug ineffective.

2. **Absorption rate:** Your genes influence how quickly drugs go to work. If your genes give you a tendency to absorb a drug very slowly, you may need either a higher dose of the drug or a different, more speedily absorbed drug.

3. **Resistance:** Some people are completely unaffected, or resistant, to certain drugs. This occurs if your genes react to the drug by manufacturing blood-borne proteins that can obstruct the drug's passage through your body, rendering it ineffective.

4. **Metabolism:** Just as some people seem to be able to eat heartily and never gain weight and others can't, different

people metabolize drugs at different rates. This somewhat unpredictable factor can make it difficult to calculate the proper dose.

5. **Elimination:** Drugs are eliminated from the body after a period of time. How long that takes is, in part, determined by your genes.

## Understand how your race may factor into your response to certain types of drugs.

In many instances race can yield clues to discovering if you have a genetic predisposition that could affect your response to a particular medication. For example, an estimated 20 to 25 percent of Asians lack the enzyme needed to break down and process diazepam, or Valium, effectively. Yet a mere 1 percent of Asians lack the enzyme needed to break down the non-steroidal anti-inflammatory drugs (NSAIDs) ibuprofen (Motrin) and naproxen (Naprosyn).

However, that particular enzyme deficiency is a common problem in treating African Americans with hypertension. Armed with this knowledge, doctors have learned to use a different approach: According to an article by Dr. W. D. Hall in the *American Family Physician* (February 1999), the first line of defense against hypertension in African Americans is the use of diuretics. So if you are an African American newly diagnosed with high blood pressure, and you are put on an NSAID, you will want to find out whether your doctor has taken into account the likelihood of a genetic predisposition when prescribing your course of treatment.

Caucasians, similarly, have difficulties with certain families of medications. About 7 percent lack the enzyme to break down codeine, for example. In the future, perhaps tests to determine the presence or absence of such an enzyme will be routine. In the meantime, your best defense is knowing whether or not any of your blood relatives have had problems with a medication, and making sure your doctor has that information before you are in a situation in which you might be given that drug.

## Report any other reason you may have for avoiding a particular drug or class of drugs.

Some people would much rather take a mild pain reliever and endure a little pain or discomfort than have hours of that "disconnected" feeling associated with strong narcotics like Vicodin or Percocet. That's perfectly legitimate—all you should need to do is inform your doctor of the fact. There are alternatives available. Most likely, you'll get a prescription for Tylenol 3 and you may even be able to get a little work done while you heal.

On the other hand you may be worried that all you will get after surgery is Tylenol 3, which you know from past experience doesn't do much for you when you're in severe pain. If you know the specific name of a drug that's worked for you in the past, by all means request it. Your doctor will tell you if it's appropriate for use in your case.

## Report all food allergies to both your doctor and your anesthesiologist.

It's not just a matter of being sure the hospital doesn't serve you strawberries which give you hives. Certain food allergies are actually warning signs of drug allergies. Take, for example, a shellfish allergy: Patients allergic to shellfish are often allergic to iodine as well. Another example of a common allergy overlap is to eggs and *propofol*, a common anesthetic. Because propofol is suspended in an egg-soy-lecithin emulsion, any patient with a true egg allergy is at risk for a bad reaction to this drug. Since propofol is used in many *intensive care units* (ICUs), it's essential, too, that all your medical caregivers are informed as soon as you know you're on your way to the hospital.

In medical emergencies when you don't have time to answer presurgical interview questions or fill out forms (or you are unconscious or otherwise physically unable to do so), you should be sure that your medical records will be accessible and that they reflect all your drug allergies and sensitivities. (For more ideas about how to make sure your medical information is accessible in an emergency, be sure to read Chapter 9, "When You Have No Time to Plan.")

## Know the dangers of taking certain herbal supplements before surgery.

If you're about to go into the hospital, particularly for surgery, one of the things you do not want to do is add herbal therapies to your dietary regimen, because of the unknown risks of interactions between medications commonly used in hospitals and whatever supplements you may be using.

As noted in the tips above, you should report any and all substances you take regularly—and that means all prescribed drugs, over-the-counter drugs, vitamins, minerals, and herbal remedies—to your doctor, either in a list or by bringing in the containers.

Herbal therapies pose a particularly thorny problem for most doctors concerned about drug interactions because the herbal drug industry is so poorly regulated, and labeling of ingredients is often vague or even deliberately misleading. It can be difficult to figure out exactly what chemicals are contained in some herbal "therapies," much less how your body will react to them while under the influence of other drugs. Under the law that presently governs the manufacture and sale of herbal products, the Dietary Supplement Health and Education Act (DSHEA) of 1994, these so-called "food supplements" do not have to undergo the same sort of rigorous testing given to pharmaceuticals, nor is their dispensing regulated by federal authorities.

In case of reported side effects or harm from the use of an herbal remedy, the burden is on the U.S. Food and Drug Administration (FDA) to prove there is a problem; the manufacturer has no responsibility to prove there's not a problem. For example, after compelling anecdotal evidence that ephedra is a health risk, the FDA commissioned a study. The results of the study conducted by clinical pharmacology scientists at the University of California at San Francisco showed that use of the herb was responsible for several cases of heart attack, stroke, and seizure. After the release of the study there was some tightening of the law regarding claims made on product labels, but labels still don't make it clear what kind of substance interactions to avoid or give any warnings about possible dangerous side effects.

Problems persist: During 1998, the Dietary Supplement Poison Center Study Group evaluated calls to ten poison control centers to find out how often people called with supplement-related adverse reactions and what those problems were. Commonly reported symptoms included gastrointestinal problems, hypersensitivity reactions, and effects on the central nervous system. A few of the cases ended in death. Among the big culprits here were ephedra (commonly marketed as the Chinese herbal ma huang), St. John's wort, kava, ginkgo, ginseng, and melaleuca oil.

Even if you have been using herbal remedies up to now without a problem, there are good reasons why you should quit before surgery. First, you cannot predict what sort of interaction may occur between the herb you take and any of the drugs used during or after surgery. Second, in your weakened condition as a surgical patient, you might experience harmful side effects from the cumulative dose of the herb in your system that your body would have tolerated quite well in its pre-surgery state of health.

To learn which herbs are particularly implicated in surgery-related drug interactions, I recommend that you log onto the Internet to view the charts compiled by Susan C. Smolinske, a doctor of pharmacology and managing director of the Regional Poison Control Center at Children's Hospital of Michigan. Of particular interest is the chart titled "Red Flag List: Dietary Supplements—Adverse Reactions," which lists 34 common dietary supplement from aconitum (aconite) to wormwood, and the known adverse reactions produced by each, including, in a few cases, heart attack, liver toxicity, renal failure, depression of breathing, and stroke. (Log onto ***http://www. mcmahonmed.com/wworks/CHARTS/herbdrug/default.html***, click on "Tables," and then click on "Table 1.")

In another chart, "Dietary Supplements—Drug Interactions," found on the same website, Dr. Smolinske also lists supplements that have been found to produce dangerous reactions when taken in combination with certain medications. (Go to the same web address as above, click on "Tables," and then click on "Table 4.") The findings on this chart provide even more detailed cautionary advice to anyone who relies on these substances or even uses them occasionally. In particular, the chart's "Anticipated Effect" column warns of interactions between certain supplements and drugs that have been found to

**What's the worst that could happen** if you mix incompatible herbs and drugs? Let me summarize a story I found in an article titled "Dietary Supplement Adverse Reactions & Interactions: 2000 Update" by Dr. Susan C. Smolinske in the June 2000 issue of *Anesthesiology News*.

A patient at Dr. Smolinske's hospital who had been taking an *angiotensin-converting enzyme (ACE) inhibitor* had a mild systemic hypersensitivity reaction after he accidentally took his wife's St. John's wort. ACE inhibitors are commonly used to reduce blood pressure by dilating blood vessels. According to Dr. Smolinske, combining ACE inhibitors with certain herbs can result in a life-threatening anaphylactic reaction. Apparently, the risk of using the herb was not made clear to him, because a few weeks later, he made the same mistake, but this time the reaction caused his death.

Dr. Smolinske goes on to note that combining another commonly used class of cardiac drugs, *beta-adrenergic block agents (beta-blockers)* with certain herbal supplements can produce the same life-threatening or even fatal results.

produce lowered respiration or blood pressure, or increases in sedation or toxicity, any of which could have severe consequences if occurring during surgery. Even a quick perusal of Dr. Smolinkse's findings underscores how important it is to let your doctor know what herbal supplements you are taking, as well as how often and how much.

Don't just make a list, either. Bring in the actual bottles or product labels. Also, ask your doctor to check with your anesthesiologist about possible reactions between supplements you've been on and the anesthetics to be used in your procedure. Once you know who will be your anesthesiologist, remember to inform him or her directly of your supplement use history. You don't want a last-minute discovery of the problem to result in your being sent home rather than risk unknown interactions. And you certainly don't want to run the risk of having surgery with any of your doctors unaware of the potential for life-threatening interactions.

**Tell your doctor if you have an allergy to rubber products, or suspect you do, and repeat that information in every interview you have prior to surgery.**

Latex allergies are becoming more common because more people are repeatedly exposed to rubber products. Latex gloves and other items are found in most hospitals and clinics, and if you are allergic to the substance, you might react by developing a rash, hives, or a headache, or even serious breathing problems. As long as there is advance notice, your surgical team will be able to avoid any ill effects by switching to latex-free equipment; they just wheel in a specially designed latex-free supply cart with the items they need—gloves, IV lines, breathing circuits, and so forth. Be aware, however, that there are some surgical facilities unable to accommodate patients who are allergic to latex. It's essential that you find out whether yours is one of them well before the date of your surgery. Should you discover that latex-free supplies are not available, you should certainly take steps to postpone your surgery and reschedule it in a facility that meets your medical needs.

**Tell both doctors and nurses about any skin sensitivities or skin conditions, and especially about past skin reactions to bandages or surgical tape.**

Most hospital procedures are rough on your skin—even if your skin is hearty and healthy. Harsh antiseptics are used to sterilize areas, bandages compress skin, tape pulls, and the adhesives irritate. But when you have sensitive skin, either because you have eczema or psoriasis or because you're older and your skin has thinned with age, you should certainly ask that extra care be taken to see that your skin is treated as gently as possible.

Tape is a particularly common problem for many patients. It's used to keep your IV line in place and perhaps to keep your eyelids shut during surgery. (Your eyelids need to stay closed so that your eyes don't dry out, which can lead to painful corneal abrasions. The alternative to tape over your eyelids is a gooey substance that seals and lubricates them.)

The simplest way to find out if you are likely to have a reaction to the tape your surgeon uses is to ask for a swatch of it. Put it on the back of your hand for a couple of hours and see if you get a reaction. If so, then request that paper tape be used whenever possible. It's usually far less irritating, although it doesn't hold as strongly as regular surgical tape.

**Make sure that everyone in your surgical team knows about any artificial implants, joints, pins, or other foreign objects inside your body.**

Most implants are made of metal. Before many surgical procedures you will first have a *magnetic resonance imaging (MRI)* test. Any metal in your body could interfere with the MRI scanning equipment; it can also cause problems in the use of electrical surgical equipment. The same is true for shrapnel or other objects that may have ended up inside you.

Even if you are not scheduled for an MRI, chances are good that your surgery will involve a *Bovie,* an electrical device used to reduce bleeding. A Bovie pad (or plate), which spreads the electrical current, goes next to your skin and needs to be placed away from any metal in your body. A Bovie pad is cold, by the way. When the nurse or doctor tells you, "This is going to be cold," you should be prepared for "ice cube."

Yet another reason to report any foreign objects in your body is comfort. If a bone screw is close the skin, for example, pressure on it could be painful. If your surgical team members know ahead of time, they can cushion the area.

**Ask your surgeon to give you a general description of what will happen during surgery.**

In Chapter 1, I suggested that you do some research to learn what you can about the procedure that you need, but that doesn't mean it's all up to you on your own. Your surgeon should definitely be asked (if he or she hasn't already volunteered) to explain, in simple, step-by-step terms, what will be happening while you're unconscious on the operating table. You're not looking to get a medical school lesson but just enough of a sense of what the procedure involves so that you don't feel helpless, overly anxious, or ignorant as you allow yourself to be "put under."

## Clear up any doubts you have about how your procedure will be performed, and why it is the best choice to deal with your medical problem.

You don't want to go in to surgery in a state of complete anxiety about whether you're doing the right thing. If, as the date approaches, you learn something that makes you wonder if another treatment would be a wiser course, by all means, bring the matter up with your surgeon. No good doctor wants to perform a procedure on a reluctant patient; an even worse consequence might be that you'd change your mind at the last minute and the scheduled procedure would have to be cancelled.

In all likelihood, your surgeon will remind you of the reasons that led you to seek him or her out to perform the procedure in the first place and put your mind at ease. If, for example, you've learned in the interim about some new procedure that seems less invasive and more promising, your surgeon should be able to answer your questions about its applicability, or lack of applicability, in your case. If your surgeon isn't able to reassure you, then seriously consider postponing your operation until you've had the chance to explore your options as thoroughly as you can and become convinced that you're doing what's right for you.

## Keep in mind: Even the best doctors don't know everything.

I'll let you in on a little professional secret: Doctors sometimes like you to believe that they know more than they do. We like to be looked up to. Some of us don't especially like to be questioned. There's a distinctive way a doctor might talk about how much he's learned in his career. If something has happened to one patient, he says it's "... in my experience." If it has happened to two patients, it's "... in my series of patients." If it has happened to three patients, it's "... in patient after patient after patient." A corollary adage many doctors rely on is: "Do something that works well for you and stick to it."

There are advantages and disadvantages to following this rule, but the underlying truth is that the doctor who does so is choosing his treatments on the basis of his own personal experience, rather than on the basis of large-scale studies done according to scientific standards. Now perhaps, if that doctor has a wealth of experience doing the particular surgery and/or using the therapies that are just right for your condition, you will be well served—in fact, better served than if you'd gone to someone who relied on abstract reading of studies.

I'll give you an example from my own field of anesthesiology: A doctor uses an anesthetic recipe that works very well in 99 percent of her patients. There is no point in changing unless a patient with a special case comes along. But a doctor with such a philosophy is also less likely to adapt to beneficial innovations and techniques. In orthopedics, for example, there's a machine that's become widely used in the last decade called a continuous passive motion machine, or CPM. Following surgery on a knee or elbow (typically), the patient's affected part is attached to the machine, which then exercises it in slow, repetitive motions. Not every orthopedist uses it, however; there are a few who stick with the same rehabilitation course they used before this machine was invented. If a patient requests the use of the new machine after surgery, the answer might be, "It's my experience that in these cases if the machine is used, a graft can come loose."

If you're that orthopedic patient told that the CPM isn't for you, I would urge you not to be intimidated by the idea that the doctor knows so much more than you do. If you have reason to wonder at something a doctor has told you, ask a follow-up question: "How many times have you seen that happen?" and "Why do you think other doctors are using the CPM after surgery?" If you still find the answers leave you unconvinced, then it's probably time to find a different doctor who can give you answers that make more sense to you.

**Make sure you are clear on exactly where you are to report for surgery and at what time.**

You don't want to show up at the hospital only to discover you have no idea where in this vast warren of departments and wings and out-buildings your procedure is to take place. Ask your doctor's office assistant for a map and a detailed set of directions so that you can know exactly where to report. If you're going by car, find out where to park, too.

And finally, you need to know what time you're supposed to be there (not what time the procedure is supposed to start, which may well be two or three hours later). Make sure that you and whoever will be accompanying you both have been told the same time, and that you both have reliable alarm clocks you can set to make sure that you're up in time to get prepared for the big event.

### Make sure you are clear on your pre-surgery instructions concerning food, use of medications, and other details. (And get all this in writing!)

In the normal course of events you will be provided with a sheet of instructions—but if you don't have one, definitely ask for it. Read it carefully while you're in the doctor's office and ask questions about anything you don't understand completely. (If you received it by fax or in the mail, then read it carefully at home and call your surgeon's office with your questions and concerns.)

Take it home and put it someplace prominent, where you'll be sure to see it on the night before surgery and the following morning, too. I'd say stick it to the door of your refrigerator with magnets, since one of your instructions will almost certainly be "Nothing to eat after midnight prior to surgery." That way, you'll see it in the morning as you absent-mindedly go for that glass of orange juice, and you'll be reminded not to open that door.

### Find out where and when you will be when the surgery is over and have a sense of what will happen next.

Most likely, you'll be in the recovery room. Ask about how long patients usually stay there before being moved to their own room. Find out if you'll be conscious, able to talk, and whether you'll be able to learn how the procedure went. Ask about how much pain most patients report feeling right after surgery (and be aware that your surgeon will probably try to avoid the word "pain" and talk instead about "discomfort.")

**Discuss with your surgeon ways to minimize the incision scar.**
After your surgery is done and the healing time is over, you want your body to look as normal as possible. That means you want the least visible scar. The look of your scar, or the apparent lack of a scar, can depend on whether your surgeon used staples or sutures to close your incision. Not only that, but different kinds of sutures can be used. Surgeons can use dissolving sutures, for example. That might take a few more minutes than closing with staples, but as far as you're concerned the result will be worth it. Plastic surgeons, who know how to disguise their handiwork as much as possible, commonly use something called a *subcuticular stitch.* This is also known as a *plastic closure* because it is so often used in plastic surgery. It takes a little longer to do—maybe three minutes—but the result is often more cosmetically appealing. If the incision will be made in any area of your body that shows when you're wearing a swimsuit, you should certainly ask about having a plastic closure.

Your race may also be a factor in the appearance of your post-surgical scar. Some people with dark skin have a tendency to form overgrown scars, known as *keloids,* which can itch and burn. A similar condition, called a *hyptertrophic scar,* is also unaesthetic but doesn't cause physical discomfort. If you have dark skin and want to reduce the risk of this prominent type of scarring, you should insist on sutures. A subcuticular stitch doesn't guarantee you a good result, but it certainly does increase the odds in your favor.

**If you are to have *nasogastric (NG) tube* in place for your surgery, or any type of catheter inserted, ask if this can be done during your surgery under general anesthesia.**
An NG tube runs from your nostril down to your stomach. Inserting it will irritate you at the least and at the worst cause you much pain. The same is true for *urinary* and *central venous catheters* as well. Sometimes the clinical situation will not permit the doctor to place the tube while you're under general anesthesia for your surgery, but

sometimes it can. In any event, you will be better off bringing the matter up with your surgeon ahead of time, so that if it is possible, it can be arranged. If you wait until your doctor or technician is approaching you with the apparatus, it might well be too late for the sequence of events to be changed.

### Look into the feasibility of donating your own blood in preparation for elective surgery.

*Self-donation of blood* (called *autologous donation*) is only practical for elective operations and when your general health permits. If your procedure carries with it some potential risk of substantial blood loss (as is the case, for example, in a prostatectomy or in a total hip replacement), you would be well-advised to put this recommendation into practice. Ask your doctor if you are a good candidate for autologous donation. If the answer is yes, your doctor should be able to help you plan the donation so your body has time to replenish its internal blood supply before the procedure. For many elective surgeries, such as facelifts and knee arthroscopies, the chance of significant blood loss is so minimal, there is no point to donating in advance of your surgery.

### If your surgery will be performed in a large medical center, it's wise to inquire about *cell saver* technology.

Cell saver technology recycles your own blood that otherwise would be lost during major surgery. Although many hospitals don't yet have it, there's certainly no harm in asking if they do and, if so, requesting that it be used. In the event that you require a blood transfusion, you avoid the risks associated with donor blood through reuse of your own blood.

### Discuss the implications of any chronic problems you might have.

Your doctor needs to be aware of any long-term health problem you have, whether or not you currently take medication for it. Examples include obesity; sleep apnea; insomnia; high blood pressure; epilepsy; heartburn, acid reflux, or gastroesophageal reflux diseases (GERD);

diabetes; asthma; heart disease; joint conditions; and any disease or condition requiring the use of corticosteroids. The tips that follow give specific recommendations for patients who fit into these categories.

## Tell your doctor if you have any circulatory problems, such as *Raynaud's disease,* or if you suspect you do.

In patients with Raynaud's disease, the small arteries in the fingers and toes don't function properly. The primary symptom is extreme sensitivity to cold in the extremities, which receive little blood flow. In a Caucasian patient, the ends of the fingers would be completely white, and when blood returns to the tips, they become purplish before assuming a normal color. Since blood oxygen is usually monitored during surgery with a device called a pulse-oximeter that clips to a fingertip, it's important for your surgical team to know if the blood flow to your fingertips is impaired in any way. The pulse oximeter can be repositioned to an earlobe or another body part unaffected by the disease.

## If you are obese, ask your doctor about the advisability of getting your weight down before elective surgery.

If you are seriously overweight, you've undoubtedly been advised to lose weight by every doctor you have ever consulted. How heavy is too heavy? A reliable guide is the federal government's body mass index (BMI): Take your weight in kilograms (your weight in pounds divided by 2.2) and divide that number by your height in meters squared (your height in inches multiplied by .0254, then squared). A healthy BMI should be between 19 and 25. If your BMI number exceeds 25, you are either a strength athlete (for example, a bodybuilder or a football player) or you are overweight.

You should know that obesity makes anesthesia surgery much more dangerous. Intubation (the placement of breathing tube in your windpipe) is generally more difficult. Cutting through inches of fat to reach a damaged joint or organ makes the surgeon work a lot harder. Even starting an IV line in an obese person is a challenge because the veins are hidden under a layer of fat. People who are too heavy, either because of fat or muscle, also tend to have problems when lying down for a long period of time. Their weight on the diaphragm diminishes breathing. A clue to the fact that this can occur is whether you experience sleep apnea (see the next tip). You should also know that excess weight can make recovery more difficult. Obese people are more susceptible to infections and pulmonary embolisms (blood clots in the lungs).

Obese people may even have diminished choices on where to have a surgery done. Some operating room tables will not support patients over a certain weight. They will also find that some doctors won't perform certain elective procedures on them because of their weight. Orthopedic surgeons, for example, don't like to perform certain knee or hip operations on obese people because their weight would inhibit their ability to do the required rehabilitation exercises. Even if an obese patient got through rehabilitation, too much weight on a replacement joint could undo the surgeon's efforts.

For these and other reasons it's generally advisable for seriously overweight patients to postpone nonessential surgery until after successful completion of a doctor-supervised or hospital-monitored weight loss program. Your doctor will advise you if you are a candidate for such a program, which would put your diet under the control of a certified dietitian or a nutritionist and might also include the services of a certified personal trainer or weight-loss support group. Being in a doctor-directed program will also prevent you from being scammed by quick-weight-loss gimmick-selling organizations and allow you to discover if your weight gain is the result of a serious physical malfunction (for example, a thyroid problem) that can be treated medically.

If you need a compelling financial reason to deal with your weight problem, consider that the *American Journal of Public Health* has determined that for every 10 percent of body weight an obese person loses, he or she saves $5,200 in lifetime health care costs.

**Tell the doctor if you've been told that you snore loudly or have sleep apnea, or if you sleep upright or use more than one pillow at night.**

All of these indicate the possibility that you have breathing problems while asleep or unconscious, and have implications for your response to anesthesia. Your surgeon and anesthesiologist will be better able to deal with any breathing problems that develop if you put them on notice that you have any of these conditions.

**If you have insomnia or even occasional sleeplessness, talk to your doctor about how best to ensure a good night's rest before surgery.**

Being well rested is an important component of your overall health, which you want to be as good as it can be prior to surgery. If you currently use a sleeping aid, make sure your doctor knows what it is and how much you take, and talk about the proper dosage to use the night before surgery. You may be told to increase the dosage on a one-time basis. If you only occasionally experience sleeplessness and do not have a prescription for sleeping pills, ask your doctor whether it's advisable for you to have the option of taking one, in the event that you find yourself too nervous too sleep the night before.

**If you have high blood pressure, discuss with your doctor how your medication-taking patterns will be affected.**

Find out whether the doctor wants you to take the medication as usual on the day of surgery, and find out whether there will be any adjustments in the first days after surgery.

**If you have epilepsy, ask the same questions as above about your anti-seizure medication.**

You especially want to be clear on whether to take a dose the same day that you have surgery.

**If you have heartburn, acid reflux or gastroesophageal reflux disease, ask the same questions as above about your antacids or acid-blocking medications.**

Your doctor may have special instructions for you about taking a nonparticulate antacid such as sodium citrate the same day of surgery and a few days afterward. For more information on this point, see Chapter 6, "Getting Ready to Go."

**If you have diabetes, your doctor may advise you to cut your insulin injection in half before surgery.**

Without any food or drink in the body, the need for insulin changes. In some cases, the insulin injection will be eliminated just before surgery. In other cases, because you will receive steroids as part of the surgical procedure, more insulin might be necessary, because steroids tend to reduce the effectiveness of insulin injections. Sometimes the surgical staff, which is monitoring your blood sugar along with other critical signs, will opt to administer insulin at some point during the procedure. It's critical that your medical care team work carefully with you to manage your condition both in the time before surgery and just afterward. So keep them completely and accurately informed about your blood sugar levels and insulin usage and follow their instructions to the letter.

**Asthma patients should always bring their inhaler to the hospital on the day of surgery.**

If you do need your inhaler but you left it at home, the hospital can take care of you—but you won't like the price.

**If you have a pacemaker, call the manufacturer about your planned surgery and take your pacemaker information card with you to the hospital.**

Every patient with a pacemaker must be issued a card that states what kind of pacemaker it is, the year it was put in, the last time the battery was changed/checked, and the toll-free number that you can call to program it over the telephone.

If you have to have surgery, sometimes a representative of the company that made the pacemaker will meet you at the hospital to ensure that it continues to function at that critical time. To take advantage of this service, you must of course see to it that the company is informed well in advance of your procedure.

**If you are on corticosteroids, check with your surgeon and/or your anesthesiologist about the dose to take on the day of surgery.**

The likelihood is that you will need a supplemental dose beforehand. If you have been using anabolic steroids—as many bodybuilders, power-lifters, football players, and other types of athletes do to build muscle mass—be sure that your doctor is aware of the fact. Steroids can cause heart, liver, or kidney damage, which could affect your anesthesia requirements as well as your surgical outcome. Even if you believe you've been using these substances safely, for your health's sake, take a break from the "juice" when you know you're headed for surgery.

**If you have a joint condition that could be aggravated by lying on a hard surface, ask about having your surgery done on a stretcher.**

For certain types of surgery—hand and foot, for example—it is possible to avoid moving from your comfortable stretcher to an operating table for the procedure. If you've found that staying on a hard surface causes you pain, then ask your doctor about this possibility.

**Come to your pre-surgery interview with your own *written* list of questions and concerns.**

No matter how much you've read up on your problem and your impending surgery, you will undoubtedly still have questions. After all, books and articles are about other people, not your own unique case. You want to hear how the doctor thinks things will go *for you*. He or she might already have briefed you and told you what you need to know. But if not, write down any questions that you think still need to be answered and give them to your doctor.

The box on page 68 lists some of the questions that you should certainly ask (unless the doctor has already answered them for you). Be sure you're clear about the answers, too. If you aren't, then follow up by asking for an explanation of any parts you found confusing.

**Take notes during your pre-surgical interview.**

It won't do you much good if the doctor has told you everything you need to know but later you find you've forgotten much of what you learned. Just as your doctor keeps notes in his or her patients' files, you should take notes when your doctor talks. And remember to bring your notes to the hospital with you. That way you won't be calling your doctor from your hospital bed to ask how much longer you can expect to have a catheter stuck in you—you can just consult your notes.

### Questions to Be Answered Before Surgery

Not all of these questions need to be fielded by your doctor. Please note that some are better handled by the doctor's support staff or by hospital nurses.

- How long do you expect the surgery to last?

- How common is it for the surgery to take longer? Why?

- How often will you be checking on me after the surgery?

- How do most patients feel afterward? Should I expect some pain?

- What kind of pain medication will I get, and how often can I expect to receive it? What do I do if the pain medicine doesn't work?

- What will my day be like after the surgery? Where will I be when I wake up? Will I be moved to my hospital room, and if so when? Will I be able to go to the bathroom?

- What will the days after that be like? Will I have tests? Therapy? What type and how often?

- When do I get to eat and drink again? Will there continue to be dietary restrictions?

- How soon after surgery will they let me see my family (mom, wife, boyfriend, other visitors)?

- Can I take a shower?

- (If you're an outpatient) What time can I leave?

**If you find the date of surgery is looming and there are still issues raised in this chapter (or in the next chapter on anesthesia) that have not been covered, either in a written pre-surgery questionnaire or in a pre-surgical interview, be persistent about getting an answer.**

Let's suppose you mentioned to your doctor that you were scheduled to have some bridgework done in the week following your cataract surgery. Somehow your question about postponing the dental work never got answered. Don't go into the hospital still worried about it. Call the doctor's office and leave the question as a message. The doctor doesn't want patients to be nervous or uncertain about anything before surgery and will surely get back to you (or have a nurse or office assistant get back to you) with the information you seek.

If both you and your doctor are computer users, a good way to get non-emergency questions asked and answered is by email. That way there's no "telephone tag," and both you and the doctor have a written record of the information given out, which can be very important if something goes amiss and there is some implication that you weren't following your doctor's orders.

# CHAPTER 4

# All About Anesthesia: How to Make Sure Your Doctor Knows What It Takes to Keep You Out of Pain

In all probability, your procedure will involve some form of anesthesia or pain control. Anesthesia is one area of medicine in which patient options have rapidly expanded while patient safety has improved dramatically. Patient deaths attributable to anesthesia have dropped from 1 in 10,000 cases in 1980 to less than 1 in 250,000 in the year 2000 (statistic reported on *NBC Nightly News,* August 15, 2001).

Nevertheless, anesthesia remains one of the most complex areas of surgical practice, calling for careful decisions to be made at every stage of your care. It's becoming commonplace in any procedure involving anesthesia to collect information from the patient specifically to aid in predicting how he or she will respond to the drugs that may be used. Although many of the questions in an interview with the anesthesiologist or on the pre-anesthesia form will duplicate those on your general health questionnaire or in your pre-surgical interview, remember that this time your answers are being reviewed by different medical team for a particular purpose—you're not just being asked the same things over again because the anesthesia team can't be bothered to look things up in your records. In fact, it's to your benefit to have this duplication of questions. You may remember to include a detail in one interview that you left out of the other, or one doctor may notice and act on some aspect of your background (for example, your reported allergy to eggs) that another doctor thought was of little consequence. By going through another pre-surgical interview, you also get the opportunity to ask more questions and become more comfortable with the nature of the operation you are going to have.

Your goal in answering the questions is to become a helpful partner in the decision-making process, an active member of the team that includes your surgeon, your anesthesiologist, the surgical assistants, and other members of the hospital staff. For this to come to pass, you need to do more than provide accurate and complete information. You also need to know something about the purpose the information serves. You need to understand your choices in pain control, both during and after your procedure. You also should know how to express your preferences and state your medical needs in a way that allows your medical caregivers to recognize and respect them.

That's what the advice in this chapter is intended to help you to do. As in the Chapter 3, you will undoubtedly find recommendations that don't apply to your situation, but pay close attention to all that do. I don't want to alarm you, but anesthesia reactions do happen, and they can be life threatening. By paying close attention to all the points in this chapter you will go a long way toward bringing the risks attendant with anesthesia down to the lowest possible level. And you will have a more comfortable experience, too.

### Understand the choices for anesthesia in your case.

We've come a long way since the days when the painkilling alternatives for a patient were an ether-soaked rag, a shot of whiskey, or biting on a bullet. Nowadays options for anesthesia cover a lot of bases: There are different drugs used for *sedation;* there are different approaches to anesthesia (that is to say, general, regional, or local, also categorized by type: e.g., *spinal, epidural, caudal, topical, nerve block*) and there are different methods for delivering the anesthesia: mask, intubation, catheter, injection, spray, cream.

*General anesthesia* entails the use of a number of different drugs, all with the effect of turning you into an unaware, immobile body. Anesthesia professionals now realize, however, that the type of anesthesia you receive can affect your dreams, substantially improving your state of mind when you wake up from sedation. To that end and for many other reasons, the most commonly used drug is now propofol. Anesthesiologists commonly ask patients who've had anesthesia if they had pleasant dreams. After propofol, patients tend to answer with a purring sort of "yes." I've even had female patients wake up from propofol and ask me to go on a date!

Don't opt for general anesthesia just for the dreams, though. When the choice of having *local* or *regional anesthesia* is an option, my bias is in favor of it because, in many cases, it's less risky than general anesthesia, as well as being less likely to bring uncomfortable side effects, such as nausea and vomiting and the feeling of loss of control.

Other compelling reasons to have local or regional anesthesia are that these forms of anesthesia often give pain relief that lasts longer than the surgery, and so you need less of other pain drugs afterward. Also, you tend to have less bleeding.

Local or regional anesthesia is *not* an option for everyone, however. You will need general anesthesia if

- The scope of the surgery is such that a local or regional anesthetic would be inadequate to the task. Most chest and abdominal operations are of this type.
- The surgeon either rarely or never performs the particular operation on semi-conscious patients.
- The patient doesn't accept the idea of being semi-conscious during surgery. Even with a regional block in place, patients still feel pressure and touch. In some cases, there is also noise associated with the procedure that can be upsetting to certain sensitive patients.

*Regional blocks* can be used to numb entire sections of the body. For a hand, fingers, or the entire lower arm, the anesthesiologist or nurse-anesthetist could do a couple of things. One is to put a tourniquet on the arm, then administer an intravenous regional block. As long as the operation is not much longer than an hour, the tourniquet shouldn't be painful. An alternative is called an *axillary block,* which involves an injection in the armpit to block the major nerves as they enter the arm. Also, there are *nerve blocks,* which are used in cases involving the ankle, groin, buttocks, and parts of the face.

One of the most common types of regional anesthesia is *spinal anesthesia,* which, when applied through the patient's back, numbs the entire lower part of the body. It works well in many procedures that involve just the lower part of the body, such as a cesarean section, hernia repair, hip and knee surgery, and transurethral resection of the prostate (TURP). Spinal anesthesia doesn't make all sensations disappear. A woman will probably feel some tugging and pressure during a cesarean section, and an orthopedic patient may feel pressure in the area where the doctor is working. For a TURP patient, spinal is the ideal anesthesia. Some of the side effects of this type of surgery may occur as a result of the washing (irrigating) solution used in the bladder; these may be: confusion, temporary fading of vision, and difficulty breathing. With the spinal, however, the patient is often awake enough to report these events.

A variant of the spinal is called *epidural anesthesia.* The epidural needle goes into the expandable space that lies between the skin and the spinal cord. This block takes hold more slowly, which actually can be an advantage in that it's less likely to produce a severe drop in blood pressure than a spinal block. Another advantage is that a small tube, or catheter, can be placed in the epidural space to allow the block to be used continuously over hours or even days, whereas a true spinal block lasts only a few hours.

Of course, a certain risk comes with any anesthetic. In the case of epidural anesthesia, relatively large amounts of the anesthetic drug are needed, which can cause serious complications if put in the wrong place. If it ends up in a vein, the anesthetic drug may cause convulsions or cardiac arrest. If it gets into the fluid surrounding the spinal cord, called the CSF, the drug may spread too high in the body and stop the patient's breathing. Obviously, the patient needs to be closely monitored as the epidural is being administered to make sure the anesthetic is being delivered to the correct spot.

*Local anesthetics* are typically used in procedures involving very limited areas of the body, such as removal of cataracts from the eyes or vision correction using specially designed lasers (LASIK surgery). In these eye procedures sometimes nothing more than anesthetic drops or numbing injections in the eye will be necessary. Removal of skin lesions, to take another example, is almost always done with just a local. A numbing solution may be sprayed on the area or an anesthetic may be injected that numbs only the wart or mole to be removed. Procedures done with only local anesthesia are usually so safe that there is less need for monitoring and are typically performed in the doctor's office or clinic.

---

***Anna made it very clear*** before her second knee surgery that she wanted to avoid general anesthesia if at all possible: "I told the anesthesiologist that my orthopedic surgeon said I would be under general, but I wanted him to be honest with me—did I have another option? 'Absolutely!' he said. 'I can give you an epidural and a sedative.' I was so grateful and relieved that I went into surgery with a much more positive attitude."

\*\*\*\*\*\*\*\*\*\*\*

***For several months in a row,*** Terry went into the hospital-based fertility clinic around the time of her ovulation to have her eggs surgically retrieved, as part of her effort to become pregnant through in vitro fertilization (IVF). Before the procedure started, she was given a shot of Versed, which made her feel quite drowsy and relaxed.

After her first egg retrieval, it had seemed to Terry as if the time had passed by in an instant. She found herself in the recovery area with no memory of ever having been anywhere else. The second time was the same. On the third attempt, Terry decided to take steps to be sure she would have some record of what had happened (this might, after all, mark an essential event in the life of her future child). She asked her husband, a journalist, to bring along a tape recorder and record the entire process, including his own conversations with the doctor as the doctor worked. Having the tape to listen to when she got home meant a lot to Terry, even when the procedure didn't result in pregnancy. Knowing what went on while she was sedated gave her a feeling of comfort and control over her own body during a terribly stressful time in her life.

---

## Risk-Benefit Comparisons

| Anesthesia Type | Method | Benefit |
|---|---|---|
| **GENERAL** | Intravenous medicine to sleep (anesthetic gases via breathing tube or mask) | Patient is unaware, unconscious; sedation not an issue because unconsciousness is achieved |
| **REGIONAL** | | |
| **Spinal** | Small needle in back to inject numbing medicine in space holding spinal fluid, usually below level of spinal cord | Numbness, lack of most sensation, perhaps less nausea and vomiting than with use of gas; patient may stay awake or be sedated |
| **Epidural** | Slightly larger needle in back than spinal to inject numbing medicine in space more superficial than spinal fluid space | Numbness, lack of most sensation, perhaps less nausea and vomiting than general anesthesia; patient may stay awake or be sedated |
| **Nerve Block** | Medicine injected to numb specific area such as the arm, leg, finger, eye, face, etc. | Patient may stay awake or be sedated; perhaps less nausea and vomiting than with general anesthesia |
| **Local with sedation or MAC (monitored anesthesia care)** | Smaller, more isolated amounts of numbing medicine used by surgeon combined with pain medicine (narcotics and sedatives such as Versed or Valium) by anesthesia team | Usually smaller amounts of local used; patient may be minimally or heavily sedated (e.g., "twilight sleep") |

## of Types of Anesthesia

| Risks | Side Effects | Special Considerations |
|---|---|---|
| Extremely rare: death, brain damage from lack of oxygen, dental injury, nerve injury, corneal abrasions, aspiration pneumonia, awareness during procedure | Nausea, vomiting, lingering drowsiness, sore throat, muscle aches | Sometimes difficult in obese people; patients with serious medical conditions (heart, lung, metabolic, etc.) at increased risk |
| Backache, nerve injury, spinal headache, infection, bleeding | Fall in blood pressure (transient), possible headache, feeling short of breath | Can be used for C-Section, excellent for surgeries below the waist, i.e., prostate, hernia, etc. |
| Backache, nerve injury, spinal headache, infection, bleeding | Fall in blood pressure (transient), possible headache, feeling short of breath | Can be used for C-Section; excellent for surgeries in chest and abdomen (for pain relief after operation) and below the waist |
| Nerve injury, overdose of local anesthetic, which may cause seizures | Confusion, seizures if inadvertently injected in bloodstream | Good for facelift, other cosmetic procedures; allows surgeon-patient dialogue |
| Rare: respiratory arrest, overdose of local | Nausea, vomiting, drowsiness after surgery | Good for breast biopsies, hernias, vasectomies, D&Cs, removal of skin lesions, minor orthopedic procedures, *e.g.,* carpal tunnel repair |

Another approach is using drugs that make you so relaxed that you barely notice what the doctor is doing. Sedative drugs commonly used for this purpose include ketamine, Valium, and Versed (which also has the advantage of being an amnestic, so that after the procedure is over, you may have no memory of having gone through it).

Frequently, these drugs are used in tandem with numbing agents, so that you become relaxed first, and then don't mind so much as the anesthesiologist makes punctures in your back to insert the epidural catheter or the spinal block. *Nitrous oxide,* or "laughing gas," is one sedative drug that is now only rarely used as the primary anesthetic.

Sedatives are generally regarded as very safe. Occasionally patients experience nausea or respiratory depression afterward, but unless you have had a bad experience with a particular sedative and wish to avoid it this time, you probably shouldn't be concerned about your doctor's sedative choice. One caution: Don't expect to be completely alert when your procedure is over. Sedatives typically leave you feeling woozy. Your anesthesiologist will warn you that you mustn't drive afterward and tell you to make arrangements for someone to take you home. I would add, don't make any big decisions while you still can feel the effects. After having any of these drugs in your system, just take it easy for the rest of the day. Let a loved one, nurse, or other helper take care of you until the effects have fully worn off.

### Understand your choices for your anesthesia care provider.

In many cases, you won't have a choice at all. If you are in an HMO, you usually have to take whichever provider your network has assigned to your case. But even if you are a member of a health plan that lets you choose your specialist in other areas, you may still find yourself without a choice when it comes to your anesthesiologist. Unlike your surgeon or obstetrician, most anesthesiologists belong to a *hospital-based specialty,* meaning that the hospital employs them directly or contracts with their group practice to provide in-hospital services. (The same is true for most radiologists, pathologists, and emergency medicine doctors.) Once a patient has scheduled an operation in a hospital with its own house specialists, the hospital will make the assignment based more on its own staffing considerations than on the specifics of your case.

However, if you look into this issue and discover that you do have a choice, by all means, exercise it wisely. A good start would be to ask your surgeon whether there is a particular anesthesiologist he or she prefers to work with in cases like yours. Surgeons often use the same anesthesiologists again and again, learning each other's style and pace in the OR. Your surgeon might choose to work with one anesthesiologist for one type of operation but another for a different type.

Some surgeons prefer a team approach, which combines the services of an anesthesiologist with those of a *certified registered nurse-anesthetist (CRNA),* that is, an RN who has received specialized advanced nursing training in the administration of anesthesia.

Whoever is the one to be responsible for the anesthesia used in your case should have the appropriate credentials. Find out the person's name as soon as he or she is assigned to your case. If the anesthesia provider is an M.D., find out about board certification or board eligibility (as described in the Chapter 1, page 10). If—as is the case in up to 65 percent of rural hospitals—you learn your anesthesia care will be solely in the hands of a CRNA, find out how many years' experience he or she has, and particularly inquire about the availability of many of the other safety features in anesthesia (such as Dantrolene) discussed in some of the sections below.

**Report any and all past experiences with anesthesia as specifically as possible (name of drug used, date, at which hospital) and especially report any adverse effects.**
Your anesthesiologist's best clues to how you will react to anesthesia come from your reactions in the past. It doesn't matter if, for example, the drug that your oral surgeon used to take out your wisdom teeth isn't the same as the drug that your anesthesiologist is planning to use when you have your bunion removed. If you threw up repeatedly afterwards, that's relevant information. Of course, if you already know from past experience that a particular form of anesthesia works well for you (let's say because you had an epidural during childbirth and it was a wonderful experience), go ahead and request that form of

anesthesia again. Your anesthesiologist will tell you whether it's suited to your case. The converse of this advice is also worth keeping in mind: If you've already had a miserable experience with the anesthesia used in some past procedure, ask whether this time you can try something different.

### Tell the anesthesiologist if you've ever had trouble being intubated.

Anesthesia has become a lot safer over the years due to the accuracy of monitors in the operating room and techniques used by anesthesia doctors and nurses. The big danger the anesthesia team still faces is the inability to ventilate (get oxygen into) certain patients properly. One commonly used method of giving an anesthetized patient air is by *intubation,* that is, putting a breathing tube in your trachea (windpipe). If this was difficult to do during any previous surgery that you had, your surgeon may have told you about the problem, or perhaps noted it in your medical records. Your anesthesiologist should have access to records of past surgeries, and you should certainly inform him or her if you suspect there is reason for concern over this issue.

### If you have no prior experience with intubation, know the conditions that may predispose you to intubation difficulties.

Make your anesthesiologist aware if you have any of the following: sleep apnea, prominent incisors (front teeth), a recessed chin, or the inability to open your mouth wide (usually a symptom of temporomandibular joint arthritis, or TMJ), or any other mouth, jaw, or throat problems. Prior radiation treatment to the head or neck could also lead to intubation difficulties.

### Tell the anesthesia team if you use more than one pillow at night.

Generally speaking, people who need to be propped up in order to sleep well tend not to tolerate lying down for prolonged periods. If you're not used to being in a prone position, you may experience breathing difficulties from the unfamiliar distribution of weight on your diaphragm. If you are very overweight, fatty tissue around your neck and throat can cause sleep apnea. Whatever the reason for your preferred sleeping position, it's worth bringing up in the interview with your anesthesiologist before surgery. If the staff still have you lying flat on your back as you are being wheeled to the OR, be sure to bring it to their attention before anesthesia begins.

### Tell the anesthesiologist about loose or chipped teeth.

Dental injuries that occur during anesthesia are one of the main causes of patient complaints and even litigation. They are relatively common in anesthesia practice because patients are usually so focused on the body part the surgeon will address, they neglect to address questions about their mouth and teeth—body areas of great importance to anesthesia professionals.

Patients have had loose teeth knocked out during intubation and aspirated them into their lungs. This is a serious injury. The bacteria from the mouth enter the lungs, and that can cause pneumonia and even more serious systemic infections, that is, infections in the bloodstream that can go to the rest of the body. Sometimes, if a tooth is really loose, the anesthesiologist will ask for permission to pull it before administering general anesthesia. That avoids the chance of the tooth getting sucked into your windpipe.

### Tell the anesthesiologist about any cosmetic dentistry you've had.

That way the anesthesiologist can take special care to avoid damaging your artificial crowns or implants. If you have invested thousands of dollars in making your teeth look perfect, there's no reason to put any of that work at risk; a word or two to your anesthesiologist is all that's needed to protect yourself. A plastic mouth guard is a simple but often effective tool in this regard. If your anesthesiologist doesn't suggest it, by all means, request one.

### Tell the anesthesiologist if you are right or left handed.

If you are right-hand dominant, an IV in your left hand will allow you to write, eat, and drink more easily. Most important, it will be easier for you to use the bathroom. Now that we're on that subject, there's another useful tip for patients contained in the story in the box below.

---

***I once had a patient*** who, just before carpal tunnel surgery on both her arms, took particular notice of the plastic clamps used to keep the drapes in place around her bed. The clamps look like small scissors. "What's that?" she asked, and I told her. "Do you mind if I have one of them?"

"I guess not. It costs about 29 cents. We probably won't miss it."

"I'll return it," she said.

"What? You want it, just keep it."

Then she cocked her head and smiled at me. "You can understand why I want it, can't you?"

"Well, no," I said.

"Look at what I'm having done." When I looked at the chart, I realized that the carpal tunnel surgeries on both hands would cause her to lose control over her fingers temporarily. She wanted the clamp to help her "take care of her hygiene," in other words, to hold toilet paper. Now this was a patient who was thinking ahead.

"Just keep it," I told her again. "Our gift."

---

### Report your reaction to different types of pain medicines, both over-the-counter and prescription.

You've undoubtedly used many different medicines to treat minor pain in the past: aspirin, ibuprofen (Motrin or Advil), acetaminophen (Tylenol) or combination products such as Excedrin (aspirin plus caffeine). For moderate to severe pain your doctor may have given you acetaminophen plus codeine (Tylenol 3), Percocet, Vicodin, or any of a number of other prescription drugs. If you had trouble tolerating any of these, found any of them ineffective, or experienced side effects (especially serious ones, such as bleeding or stomach distress), be sure to inform your anesthesiologist. This information will certainly figure into the selection of the right pain medication for you.

### Report your reactions to sleeping pills, sedatives, and other narcotic drugs.

Sometimes, doctors need to reverse the sedative effects of anesthesia and they do it with a drug called romazicon. This drug may precipitate seizures in people who have been long-term users of Valium or Halcion (benzodiazepines) to counter insomnia or reduce anxiety. Some people who regularly take sleeping pills or other narcotics (such as the ones mentioned in the tip above) can become resistant to the usual doses. On the other hand, there are patients who seldom take strong medications, for whom the usual dose produces an overwhelming result. In any case, it's important for your anesthesiologist to have your own account of your response in order to figure out your safest, most effective dose.

### Report your use of alcohol and your reaction to it.

Some people—especially those of small build—can get drunk from a single glass of wine. If you're one of these alcohol-sensitive drinkers, you should make your anesthesiologist aware of the fact. Instead of giving you an automatic one milligram of a sedative based on your weight, the doctor might start off with a half milligram and gauge your response before administering more. Conversely, if you regularly belt down a few stiff drinks without apparently feeling a thing (and I won't stop here to go into all the things alcohol does to you that may not be apparent), you might need more anesthesia than the average person, regardless of your weight.

Over the years, I've encountered some people who are surprisingly resistant to the effects of anesthesia. I recall a little old lady who tippled the sherry nightly needing the same anesthesia as a large, teetotaling man.

**Be frank about any substance abuse problems you may have (or may have been told you have).**

If you regularly use some substance to get high, your anesthesiologist needs to know about it, whether or not you believe you have a problem. Be assured that everyone on your medical team will hold anything you tell them in confidence, but also be clear on the point that it's necessary for them to be fully informed about anything and everything that you use that could affect your reaction to the anesthetics to be used in your procedure.

> ***When Sharon visited her boyfriend*** in the cardiac care unit, she knew that his heart attack had been set off by his cocaine use: "I said, 'Bob, have you told your doctor about your addiction?' He said, 'No' and that he had no intention of telling him. I was really torn between respecting his privacy and trying to help him get the best care. Ultimately, I decided not to say anything. I guess I made the right decision to mind my own business, but I wish he'd had the guts to trust his doctor. He never kicked the drug and ended up in the CCU all over again."

**Ask your relatives who've had surgery under anesthesia to tell you about their experiences, and especially if anything out of ordinary happened.**

If you've never been put under anesthesia before, then your best source of clues as to how you might react is to be found in the reactions of your closest relations, especially your parents. *Malignant hyperthermia* is just one several responses to anesthetic medication that has been know to run in families. This is a potentially deadly condition that occurs upon exposure to certain combinations of anesthetics. When MH is triggered, high fever, muscle rigidity, changes in vital signs, and even death can result.

Another inherited problem is deficiency of the enzyme that breaks down *succinylcholine,* a short-acting muscle relaxant. This deficiency prolongs the paralyzing effect of a certain muscle relaxant. A patient afflicted with this condition might emerge from a successful surgery only to spend days completely immobile and on a ventilator. Eventually the succinylcholine will wear off and the patient will recover, but of course it is far better to take preventive steps and avoid the situation, if family history leads you to suspect a problem.

**Fully report all substances you take, including prescription drugs, over-the-counter drugs, vitamins, minerals, other food supplements, and herbal remedies.**

Just as your surgeon needs to know what's been going into your body in order to protect you against adverse drug interactions, so does your anesthesiologist. Follow the advice on page 48 of Chapter 3 about making a complete list or bringing in the actual containers of what you take.

Be sure to note all the cautions in Chapter 3 about the use of herbal products that can interfere with anesthesia drugs.

Some "weight loss" herbal products such as ephedra, a central nervous system stimulant, can raise blood pressure and pulse rate. The use of ephedra, particularly in conjunction with other stimulants such as caffeine, has been linked to heart attacks, strokes, and seizures, according to a major study conducted at the University of California at San Francisco by Drs. Neal Benowitz and Christine A. Haller. When potent but unpredictable chemicals contained in herbal products are combined with the even more potent chemicals used in modern anesthesia, you could end up with a recipe for disaster. This warning applies equally to many other substances, including St. John's wort, which is now widely taken as a "natural" remedy for depression. For more detail on dangerous interactions between herbal remedies and pharmaceuticals, visit the website chart recommended in Chapter 3, *www.mcmahonmed.com/wworks/CHARTS/herbdrug/default.html*.

**Report all allergies and sensitivities to foods, drugs, plants, insects, and materials such as latex and adhesives.**

The reasons for doing so are given in Chapter 3. You need to repeat your account of each type of allergy or sensitivity to your anesthesiologist, to be sure he or she has the information to consider when deciding upon the type and method of anesthesia to be used. *Never assume that your surgeon will make sure that your anesthesiologist has all the essential facts.* They may work together often and have good lines of communication … or they may not. If they do, then by duplicating the information, you give your anesthesiologist a chance to question any discrepancies between one account and the other and clear up any confusion; if they don't, then you have provided essential information that your anesthesiologist didn't have before.

**Ask your anesthesiologist if your brain waves will be monitored while you are under general anesthesia to detect awareness under anesthesia.**

Once you are under a general anesthetic, you can't speak, of course, and so you have no way of communicating with your anesthesiologist if you still can feel pain. This circumstance, called *awareness under anesthesia,* is extremely rare, but it can happen, and it is devastating to the patient when it does. I tell you about it here not to scare you but to alert you to ask the anesthesia department in advance whether or not the OR is equipped with a *bispectral index system (BIS),* which monitors your brain waves to determine how anesthetized you are.

On a more reassuring note, let me add that it is perfectly normal for patients to experience some awareness of being in the operating room as they are being put under and as they are waking up.

**If inhaled anesthetics will be used, find out whether your anesthesia team has access to dantrolene to treat a potentially life-threatening reaction.**

In rare cases, inhaled anesthesia will trigger malignant hyperthermia, a reaction to the muscle relaxant succinylcholine in combination with certain inhaled anesthetics, which is characterized by high fever and hyper-metabolism. One drug will save your life when that happens—dantrolene—and not every hospital, clinic, and outpatient facility stocks it. Although this reaction occurs in only about one in every 20,000 cases, I think it's crucial that freestanding surgery centers, as well as hospitals, keep an adequate, in-date supply of this potentially lifesaving drug, which has a shelf life of three years. Malignant hyperthermia can kill, and dantrolene is the only antidote. If your procedure is planned to take place in a facility that does not stock dantrolene, I would strongly recommend that you postpone your procedure and have it moved to one that does.

### Tell your anesthesiologist if you easily become nauseated, seasick or carsick.

Anesthesia stimulates certain centers in the brain—the *chemoreceptor trigger zone.* This part of the brain is sensitive to neurotransmitters that are released during stress, pain, and motion, so patients who are prone to maladies such as seasickness and carsickness are especially likely to suffer nausea after surgery. If this description applies to you, be sure to go on to the next two tips after this.

### Ask about the use of the anti-nausea device, ReliefBand.

In 2000 the FDA approved the use of a wristband device that has had remarkable results at reducing or eliminating nausea in patients in a wide variety of circumstances, including pregnant women with morning sickness, chemotherapy patients, and post-surgical patients. In well-run, large-scale clinical trials ReliefBand has been shown to be safe, effective, and virtually without side effects (except for some possible tingling in the fingertips). As a motion sickness treatment, it's available without a prescription at many pharmacies, by catalog, or direct from the manufacturer (for contact information, see the box below). If your doctor prescribes it, your insurance company will

---

***To place a direct order*** for a ReliefBand, go to the Internet address ***www.reliefband.com*** and click on the tab marked "ordering information." You may also contact the company at 1915 Aston Avenue, Carlsbad, CA 92008, telephone: 760-804-6900, fax: 760-804-6925. To email the company for product information and general questions, the address is rbinfo@woodsidebiomedical.com.

usually pick up part of the cost, and the base cost will be lower, as well.

## Ask about getting the anti-nausea "cocktail" before surgery.

There are effective medications given before and during surgery that can prevent nausea after surgery in the great majority of patients. The one in use most often is a *"cocktail" of three drugs* that I administer to patients before they wake up, so the effects take hold before they regain consciousness and start to respond physically and emotionally to the side effects of the anesthetics. The cocktail combines Reglan (metoclopramide), which helps prevent nausea; Tagamet (cimetidine), which blocks secretion of acid from the stomach; and Zofran (ondansetron), which acts through seratonin to block the chemical responses in the brain that lead to nausea. These drugs are considered safe and usually have no side effects. The next generation of this cocktail or its components may be in the form of a small tab that dissolves under the tongue.

## Insist that the anesthesiologist or nurse-anesthetist use local anesthesia to start your IV.

Let's change the way intravenous (IV) lines enter a patient's body in this country. I have had countless patients look at me and say, "I am so scared of the IV! It hurts so bad. It frightens me more than the surgery." With the application of a local anesthetic called lidocaine this is a completely avoidable pain. To numb the skin instantaneously, the doctor or nurse will inject the lidocaine with a tiny needle that patients don't even feel.

Patients are so relieved—they often wonder why the nurses and technicians drawing their blood in the ward don't use the same local anesthesia first. For patients who are fearful about being stuck by a needle or in need of multiple tests requiring blood samples, a quick lidocaine injection should always be an option.

If you ask for one under those circumstances, your nurse might argue that she isn't trained or allowed to administer lidocaine, which is an anti-arrhythmic drug (that is, a drug that used to counter an irregular heartbeat). The counter argument to that, in my professional opinion, is that the hospital's policy needs changing. Doctors can and should train nurses to administer this local anesthesia. The required amount is so tiny—half a cc (which stands for cubic centimeter, the dosage unit for many medications)—that there is an extremely low probability of any unwanted side effects.

### Tell the doctor or nurse if you have a fear of "the mask."

Some patients see an oxygen mask coming toward them and panic. It makes them feel claustrophobic, or perhaps they're shaken by what it represents. If you are one of these people, don't be ashamed—ask for the gentle, reassuring touch you need. Perhaps it would help if the doctor or nurse could hold the mask above your face. If even that seems threatening, then your best option is to ask to have the mask removed from the tube entirely, have the oxygen output turned all the way up, and ask to be allowed to hold the tube yourself.

### Learn about your options for post-operative pain control, both in the hospital and at home.

Although your surgeon will be knowledgeable about pain control during recovery and will work closely with the anesthesiologist, I'd say you should bring your concerns and questions directly to the anesthesiologist, who is the true expert in this field. Let him or her be the one to work with you to come up with an approach to post-operative pain control that best suits your medical, emotional, and physical needs. The tips that follow describe the range of options in use in most hospitals today and tell a little bit about how they work. If your anesthesiologist doesn't discuss one of them with you, by all means bring up that technique yourself and ask if its use would be suitable in your case.

### Learn about the use of PCA and ENA devices for post-operative pain control.

The old ways to treat pain—narcotic pills and shots—are still used widely, but more and more, they are being replaced with better, more sophisticated and effective methods that insurance companies are now usually willing to cover: *patient controlled analgesia (PCA)* and *epidural narcotic administration (ENA)*.

Doctors and nurses use PCA and ENA devices on patients staying in the hospital after surgery, or on other inpatients, because the devices require monitoring and thus would be impractical for most outpatients. Examples of surgeries after which either PCA or ENA might be appropriate include hip replacement and complicated prostate surgery, both of which can cause continuous pain for many days.

The concept behind PCA and ENA is simple: Local anesthetics, like the Novocain your dentist gives and the more powerful narcotic painkillers, are administered in metered doses over the course of hours or even days. A thin tube inserted in your body is hooked up to a small computer (about the size of a cell phone) containing a cartridge that keeps dispensing drugs to block, moderate, or otherwise control the pain-transmitting chemicals being produced by your body. The PCA pump delivers the medicines into your IV line and then to your bloodstream. The ENA pump infuses the medicine through a tiny plastic tube called an *epidural catheter* near the nerve roots that emerge from your spinal cord. The ENA is used mainly for surgeries below the waist.

PCA and ENA are better than intermittent shots or pills because the concentration of drugs needed to control pain is achieved more steadily and more predictably; the peaks and valleys associated with shots and pills given at regular intervals are avoided.

Other advantages to PCA and ENA are:

- You don't have to call the nurse for pain medicine. No more repeated cries of "Is it time for my next pain shot?"
- PCA allows you to control how often pain medicine is administered. You just press a button on the small device at your side.
- You don't have to get painful injections through the skin.
- You're likely to use less medication than with oral painkillers.

For a side-by-side comparison of the PCA and ENA, see the box on page 91.

| Patient Controlled Analgesia (PCA) | Epidural Narcotic Administration (ENA) |
|---|---|
| Designed for patients staying overnight in the hospital. | Designed for patients staying overnight in the hospital. |
| Involves putting narcotic pain medication into your IV catheter, which leads directly into your bloodstream. | Involves infusing a combination of local anesthetics and narcotics through an epidural catheter, which concentrates the pain medicine close to the nerve roots of the spinal cord. |
| Can help adults control pain after almost any type of surgery. | Can control pain following abdominal surgery and other operations below the waist; epidural catheters can be placed in the thoracic spine area to give pain relief after surgeries in the chest cavity. |
| Is controlled by you with the use of a button attached to a cord. | Is controlled by an automatic computer. |
| Allows you to dictate when you need pain relief, and how much you need. | Is pre-programmed by the anesthesiologist. Doses may need to be readjusted. |
| Eliminates the need for you to call the nurse to get pain medication. | Allows the pain medicine to be infused automatically by computer, so you don't have to call the nurse. |
| Is less painful than older methods to control pain, because you don't need injections through your skin. | Is less painful than older methods to control pain, because you don't need injections through your skin. |
| Prevents you from overdosing yourself with narcotics, because there is a built-in safety mechanism that automatically turns off the infusion of medicine at a preset limit. | Prevents you from overdosing yourself with narcotics, because there is a built-in safety mechanism that automatically turns off the infusion of medicine at a preset limit. |
| Enables you to reduce side effects of narcotic use if they occur (such as itching, nausea, vomiting, and/or urinary retention) simply by pressing the button less frequently. | Can cause the same side effects found with PCA use, but the metered amount can be reduced so the side effects are consistently lowered. |

**Understand the side effects of commonly used analgesic drugs.**
In addition to different delivery methods—by injection, by pill, or by
PCA or ENA—take into account the various side effects of different
medications when considering which one might work best for you:

- *Narcotics* include Demerol, codeine, Percodan, and many
  others. Side effects can include urinary retention, nausea and
  vomiting, itching, constipation, and difficulty breathing.
- *Nonsteroidal anti-inflammatory drugs (NSAIDs)* include
  many common medications such as aspirin, Naprosyn, and
  Motrin, as well as ketorolac, which is used during surgery.
  These don't usually cause the side effects of narcotics, but
  they can be associated with ulceration, bleeding, and kidney
  damage. Also keep in mind that these side effects usually
  increase with the dose of the drug, duration of therapy, and
  patient's age.
- *COX-2 (cyclooxygenase-2) inhibitors* are a newer class of
  drugs without many of the side effects that "ruin the
  experience" of the other drugs. The ones currently
  available—celecoxib (brand name Celebrex) and rofecoxib
  (brand name Vioxx)—are given in oral form. Celecoxib is
  used to relieve osteoarthritis and adult rheumatoid arthritis;
  rofecoxib is used to relieve osteoarthritis. Both are used to
  manage acute pain.

**Consider non-pharmalogical techniques to relieve pain.**
Supplemental non-drug pain control methods, such as meditation and
the use of music in relaxation therapy, should not be overlooked. If
you have training in the use of any "mind-body" techniques and have
found them helpful in the past, by all means include them as part of
your post-surgery pain control arsenal.

**Get answers to your questions about anesthesia and
pain control.**
If you've completed your pre-anesthesia questionnaire and/or had your
consultation with the anesthesiologist but you still have questions or

concerns, call the anesthesiologist's office and ask to be called back with the information you seek. (If you know that your anesthesiologist regularly checks and responds to email, a good alternative is to send your written questions over the Internet, along with the date by which you need a response.) Before you go into surgery, you might consider asking some or all of the following questions:

- Where will I be when I wake up?
- How much pain do patients after this surgery typically experience?
- What aftereffects of the anesthesia should I expect?
- What about the sore throat that I've heard is common after intubation? Is there anything you recommend that I do for it? (Also, see Chapter 7, "In the Hospital," for my own recommendation for post-anesthesia sore throat.)
- Once I'm out of the recovery room, what pain control method will I be using?
- What are the advantages of this method of pain control as opposed to other choices?
- How will my pain medication be given? Pills? Shots? Or by one of those new patient-controlled, continuous pain medication delivery devices?
- Is this medication you recommend standard—that is, my insurance company won't fuss about paying for it—or should I be looking into getting coverage for it now?
- If my insurance company has a problem with it, can you provide me with any documentation that would help me get it covered?
- Whom should I call if the pain control method doesn't seem to be working well?

# CHAPTER 5

# Taking Care of Business: Insurance, Advance Care Health Directives, Wills, and Other Matters

Now you've done the best you can do to find the very best surgeon around, and you've made sure that your procedure will be carried out in the number one hospital in your area; you've done everything possible to be sure your surgeon and anesthesiologist know everything there is to know about your health history and other factors affecting your care—and so now it's time to learn about some things that other people can do for you. The people I'm talking about are the ones who will be helping you out when you are too weak or too "out of it" to speak for yourself. One of these people is your **patient advocate,** a person you designate ahead of time, whom you'll read about in the very first tip in this chapter. Another is your insurance company representative, who (you hope) will be taking care of the medical bills flowing out of your hospitalization, so that you don't have to worry about them. You may also wish to designate someone to express your medical wishes in the event things turn out so badly that you become incapable of making decisions for yourself—though this isn't something anyone likes to contemplate.

What all three of these people can do to help you, and many other issues besides, will be addressed in this chapter.

**Choose your personal patient advocate to watch out for your interests while you are in the hospital.**
When you are in the hospital, you might be completely incapacitated, or you might be in a somewhat weakened condition, or you might be

just slightly less than at the top of your form. However you fare, you will not be in the best shape to do a lot of arguing to get what you need. Knowing that ahead of time, you can look for someone who will take on the temporary role of your defender and champion. The person who agrees to do this for you is your designated patient advocate. If you are married, the logical choice for the role would be your spouse, who, after all, vowed to stand by you "in sickness and in health." A "significant other" who agrees to become your patient advocate is telling you by this action that he or she is truly committed to your welfare.

If you're not currently in a strong relationship, turn to your best friend or your closest family member (in your local area) to see if that person is willing to step into the role. The patient advocate must be available to accompany you to the hospital and spend a fair amount of time there with you. The person should be ready to ask questions, relay your needs to hospital staff members and doctors, and take instructions related to your care.

Once you've found the right person for the job, make sure you inform your surgeon and other doctors involved in your case, and fill in the person's name, address, phone numbers, and other contact information on the "Emergency Contact" part of all forms that you fill out before your admission to the hospital.

You should also keep a card in your wallet marked "Emergency Contact" with the person's name and phone numbers, because accidents do happen, and you never know when you might end up in the hospital without the ability to plan ahead. For a sample of what this emergency contact card should look like, see Appendix A on page 257.

**Brief your patient advocate in advance about the kinds of problems and other matters you want him or her to handle for you.**
Your patient advocate should be brought up to speed on

- what you've learned about your procedure
- where to report on the day of surgery, including where to park (if arriving by car)

- where to wait while the procedure is going on
- about how long the procedure is expected to take
- when your patient advocate can expect to see you after surgery
- whether you will be able to talk after surgery
- when you will be taken to a hospital room
- what sort of room you expect to get
- about how long you expect to stay in the hospital
- what types of medications you expect to be given, when, and what dosages (if you know or can find out ahead of time)
- any special dietary requirements the hospital is expected to meet
- any special services or extra care (such as a visit from your clergy) that you would like your patient advocate to arrange
- any matters at home you've asked your patient advocate to manage (such as watering your plants, walking your dog, bringing you your mail, making sure your bills get paid)
- any other matters that you will be unable to handle yourself while hospitalized.

**Prepare your patient advocate to intervene on your behalf whenever something in the hospital does not go according to your expectations.**
That means, if you were expecting a private room and you end up in a double, your patient advocate must go down to the admitting desk or up to the nurses' station (or both, to check whether one or the other has the greater degree of influence over the matter) to ask why you didn't receive the requested single and find out what can be done to correct the situation as quickly as possible. It helps if the person you have chosen is persistent but not hot-headed or easily rattled. The person must also have the time and energy to put in on your behalf. Of course, if you have someone willing to play this role for you, you should be sure to offer to return the favor if ever that person is hospitalized and you are well.

**Make sure both you and your patient advocate know as much as you can about the medications you'll be receiving in the hospital.**

Ask for help from doctors, nurses, or other staff members so that you will be familiar with the names and shapes of any pills you will be taking. Learn the names of drugs that will be administered through your IV drip or by injection and see if you can find out the schedule for administration of those drugs. Review all this information with your patient advocate before you are admitted. Armed with this knowledge, you will have gone a long way toward preventing medication errors, one of the most common types of bad hospital experiences. The tip in Chapter 7, "In the Hospital," page 151 is a follow-up tip giving further instruction on putting this recommendation into practice.

**Find out if the hospital has its own Office of Patient Advocacy and get to know those office staff members and what they do.**

This recommendation is not intended to become a substitute for recruiting your own patient advocate, a relative or friend who will be with you and can act on your behalf while you are at less than full energy and capabilities. It's instead a recommendation that you make use of additional resources that may be at your disposal. Many hospital administrators have become aware that medicine as it's usually practiced in large facilities these days can be faceless, intimidating, and fraught with bureaucratic rules. In order to help patients navigate through this unfamiliar maze, some hospitals have created a job of patient advocate (in larger hospitals, it's not a single job, but an office staffed with several administrators who are called patient advocates), to whom patients can complain when something goes wrong. The only trouble is, if you are feeling weak and uncertain and possibly unable to speak, you can't take advantage of the hospital's patient advocacy services. That's why you need your own personal watchdog who will look out for your interests when you can't do the job well yourself. Then, if you are in a hospital that has its own Office of Patient Advocacy, your own advocate can file complaints for you and work with the hospital's patient advocate to correct problems and make your hospital stay as good as it can be.

If your hospital does not have such an office, and you experience problems that you or your own patient advocate can't easily resolve, you might consider using the resources of an outside organization. The Patient Advocate Foundation is a nonprofit group created to help patients solve problems stemming from insurance coverage, debt management, and other crises arising from their medical care. You can contact this organization by telephone at 800-532-5274 or by email at help@patientadvocate.org, or by writing to the Patient Advocate Foundation, 753 Thimble Shoals Blvd, Suite B, Newport News, VA 23606.

**Notify your insurance company before you go to the hospital.**
Most insurance plans require you to do this before they will authorize coverage for your surgery and treatments. Many plans even dictate the hospital and specialist that you must use to be covered. Even in emergency admissions, you (or someone who can speak for you) will usually be required to inform the insurance company of your hospitalization. You may find (as pointed out below) that your surgeon's office routinely takes care of the required insurance notification for patients. But if they don't, you must be sure to take care of this essential step yourself.

**Know what your insurance covers and what's excluded.**
The time to review your insurance coverage is the day you find out you're going to have surgery. Support staff in your surgeon's office should be able to assist you in understanding what your policy provides. They will probably also take care of the required notification to your insurance company that the surgery has been scheduled and make sure you are "certified"—that is, approved for coverage. If your surgery is utterly standard, using tried and true techniques and medications, you have nothing to worry about. However, if there is anything innovative or experimental involved in the procedure, chances are your insurance company will invoke an exclusion. If you discover that to be the case in your surgery, you'll be interested in the next nine tips that follow.

## Understand insurance terms, like "experimental" and "ordinary standard of care."

Although your surgeon's office staff should be used to working with patients and their insurance companies, you'll be at an advantage if you gain some familiarity with the jargon you encounter as you check your policy and prepare forms to be submitted. There are some good books by consumer advocates on the subject. You might try reading *Making Them Pay: How to Get the Most from Health Insurance and Managed Care* by Rhonda D. Orin (Griffin Trade Paperback), *Lerner's Consumer Guide to Health Care* by Paul and Julie Lerner (paperback from Lerner Communications, Ltd.), or *Understanding Health Insurance* by Darlene Brill (a CliffsNotes booklet from Hungry Minds, Inc.). All are available online at Amazon.com.

## Challenge exclusions ahead of time, if possible.

Once you're told that some part of your procedure is excluded, you've got some work ahead of you. Even if you're rich enough not to have to worry about how you'll afford the expense, you still want to see to it that your health insurance does what it's supposed to do: Pay for the medical treatment you need. After all, that's why you've been paying those exorbitant premiums all along. So waste no time and start calling higher-ups in the company. Don't get stuck in a circular argument with the low-level person who initially turned down your request for coverage. The tip below continues this advice in more detail.

## Find out who are the right people in your insurance company to deal with—and make sure your patient advocate has their names, titles, phone numbers, and addresses, too.

You don't want to be given the runaround. Each time you deal with someone at your insurance company, make sure you get the person's name, office phone number and extension, title, and office address, and note the time and date of the conversation. Keep good records of conversations you've had and make sure that your follow-up correspondence goes to the right person. If your telephone negotiations do not resolve matters to your satisfaction, follow up by getting the name, title, and other contact information for the person who supervises that person (or someone even higher up, who has the power to reverse the previous person's decision) and appeal to that person by telephone or letter.

### Follow some simple rules in dealing with insurance company officials.

- Always be polite.
- Refrain from losing your temper, no matter what the provocation.
- Have your account number, ID number and group policy number in front of you.
- Have doctors' names, phone and fax numbers, addresses, dates of consultations, and procedure codes (if possible) at hand.
- Take detailed telephone notes during each conversation you have with a company representative, being sure to record dates and times.
- If any promises are made to you about coverage, ask that they be put in writing.
- Follow up with letters to make sure your own position is set down on paper and to get the company to respond to you in writing, either granting your request (victory!) or turning you down officially and thus providing you with a written rationale for their decision that you can appeal.

### If you have no time to challenge exclusions before you go to the hospital, prepare to pay out of pocket, but keep meticulous records to support your appeal for reimbursement.

Wouldn't you rather go into debt for a treatment that saves your life or your hearing or one of your limbs than experience the opposite outcome? Keep your health and well-being in perspective: They're far more important than your bank balance. Never allow your insurance company to outrank your doctor or make irreversible decisions about your body. Remember, you can always appeal the insurance company's ruling after you get out of the hospital, when you're well enough to take them on. But if you never regain your health because you missed your chance to have the surgery when you needed it most, you've lost something much more precious than money. So go ahead, schedule your surgery without insurance approval if you must, but save all medical diagnoses, treatment orders, lab results, bills, and other documents that you'll need to fight for the reimbursement you deserve.

**Ask your surgeon or other doctors to send letters and other medical evidence to your insurance company supporting your case for reimbursement.**

If your surgeon believes in the diagnosis he made and the treatment prescribed for you, then he ought to be willing to back up those actions with the evidence your insurance company will want to see in your appeal. He certainly should be willing to write a letter on your behalf explaining why the treatment you underwent was medically necessary and the best of all the available medical options in your case. If the exclusion was on the grounds that the treatment is unproven or experimental, he should submit any studies or other documentation he can gather showing that the use of the treatment is now so widespread as to be considered standard. Alternatively, he should submit evidence that the treatment, although not yet standard, still represented your best hope of a cure, and that no other option held out as much promise in your case.

**Set up a logical filing system for all bills, receipts, insurance forms, diagnosis sheets, lab results, and other medical paperwork. Don't throw anything out!**

This will prove useful if any of the following three events occurs:

1. The hospital overcharges you or makes other mistakes in your bill. This is actually quite commonplace: A recent study found that up to 20 percent of hospital bills are fraught with error—either overcharging or charging for services never performed. When your bills are filed systematically, it's easier for you or your financial advisor to review them for error.

2. You need to appeal an insurance exclusion. You cannot be reimbursed in the proper amount unless you have retained the proof of the amounts expended for your care.

3. You have grounds for complaint or a charge of malpractice against either the doctor or the hospital or both. To succeed with almost any kind of complaint or malpractice claim, you must be able to substantiate your account of what treatments you received, by whom, on what dates, and for what purposes—all facts supported by the bills and other medical documents saved in your files.

**Keep a log of all physicians, consultants, medical testing personnel, and laboratories that bill for services in your case.**
When you are in a busy hospital, particularly a teaching hospital, the cast of characters in your personal drama seems enormous. Keeping a running tally of who saw you, and when, can help keep you sane. Whenever you see a new face, note the name on the badge, and ask the person where he or she fits in the scheme of your care. Find out if the person is working with your private doctor, on staff at the hospital, or rotating through the hospital on the way to somewhere else.

The basic information on your list—whether you keep it in your head or on paper—could also help you answer questions like "Who set your continuous passive motion machine on three?" If you can say, "Judi Jones, the physical therapist on duty at noon," it's much more useful than "Some woman in a white coat who came in around lunchtime."

**Give the hospital's billing office the name and phone number of the person who will be handling your bills.**
The billing office won't hesitate to call you right after surgery if they have a question or problem with your insurance. You don't want to be worrying about this in the recovery room, so make sure that you have someone you can trust to look after your financial interests while you're not up to the job. This could be your designated patient advocate, or it could be someone else picked for professional expertise— your family lawyer, financial advisor, or accountant, or some other

trusted person to whom you've given financial authority. Make sure the hospital billing office knows that this is the person to call for the time being—and not you while you have a naso-gastric tube stuck down your throat.

## Make a will.
All right, you're an adult, and you know you should have done this years ago, when you first found yourself acquiring some assets and assuming some real-world responsibilities. Going to the hospital, especially for surgery, should give you the impetus you need to take care of this duty. If you own a lot, or have complicated relationships with your heirs or other potential claimants on your estate, then you'll want to use a lawyer to assist you. If you live simply and enjoy straightforward and cordial family relationships, then you may do just as well to use a template of a standard will, available in many legal software programs for your computer. (For a specific recommendation, see the tip on page 105, about advance health care directives.)

## Establish an advance health care directive.
The advance health care directive is a legal document that allows you to make your wishes known concerning the use of "heroic measures" to save your life, and what may or may not be done on your behalf should you become incompetent to make your own decisions. It should also specify who can speak for you under certain circumstances about which treatment that doctors may try to save your life and which ones you wish to be withheld.

Particularly if you are seriously ill and contemplating end-of-life issues, you will want to consider whether to include a "do not resuscitate" (DNR) order under circumstances in which resuscitation would only prolong suffering without hope of recovery. If that's your intention, then write the order unambiguously in your advance health care directive and *make sure that your family, your doctors, and hospital officials have copies of that document.*

When a doctor knows that there is a verified DNR order, then if your heart fails, you will not be subject to any lifesaving attempts of an invasive nature. Most likely, your doctor will take only those steps to end pain and keep you comfortable—a shot of morphine, for example.

One way to make your intentions clear is to express them in the "code status" jargon familiar to hospital staff. *Code Blue* treatment means that you would receive cardiopulmonary resuscitation and possibly electrical intervention—shock—and chemicals like IV drugs to help save your life. In other words, the hospital staff pulls out all the stops. A "No Code Blue" order means that you *don't* want these interventions. Write "Follow Code Blue" protocols if you do. In some cases patients want only "chemical code," that is, drugs but not shock. Your advance health care directive needs to spell out as specifically as possible what interventions you do and do not want.

---

**My late sister, Lisa,** gave an advance health care directive that resulted in her death at the age of 26. She had severe diabetes, which caused multiple complications—blindness, kidney failure, and much more.

One day, she showed up at the Catholic hospital where our father was on staff. She had a paper in her hand—her directive. She said, "I'm here to die. I don't want my insulin. I don't want you to treat me with anything but pain medicine. Here is the document that expresses my wishes. I'll probably be dead in four days."

Checking into the hospital enabled her to die in comfort and with dignity. She had prepared her family for her actions. The hospital honored her directive, and so came an end to her private hell. I often reflect on the courage and the grace of her final stand.

---

### Use a computer program to help you create legally binding documents.

The Quicken "Family Lawyer" software produced by Parsons Technology (which can be downloaded from *www.parsonstech.com*) contains guidelines on producing your advance health care directive in accordance with the law in the different states. Generally, this document consists of the elements discussed below:

**Power of Attorney for health care.** In this section you have the option of naming the responsible person and an alternate person who can make health care decisions on your behalf. If you want, you can even use the form to say that the person is authorized to make those decisions for you now, while you are still conscious and able to make them yourself. Unless you specifically limit the authority of the person you designate—and you would do that on the form—he or she can make the entire range of choices regarding your care: medical treatments, services, procedures, diagnostic tests, choice of doctors and hospitals, medications, etc. If it comes to last-resort efforts to sustain your life with artificial nutrition or cardiopulmonary resuscitation (CPR), that person can make the call to proceed or stop. That full range of authority even includes organ donations, authorizing an autopsy, and disposing of your remains. Unless you place an expiration date or end condition on the person's authority, the power of attorney goes on indefinitely. You may wish to keep it in effect, for example, until you are discharged from the hospital, or limit the effective time to those occasions when you are unable to speak or clearly signal your own intent. If you do set an ending date, keep in mind that you would have to execute a brand new power of attorney for health care the next time you need one.

**Instructions for your health care.** Whether or not you authorize another person to speak for you, you can express your own wishes regarding end-of-life decisions, artificial nutrition and hydration, and relief from pain.

**Donations of organs at death.** You can choose to donate your organs for any or all of the following purposes: education, research, therapy, and transplantation, or you can reject the idea of organ donation entirely. You can also specify certain organs to be donated but not others—for example, you could donate your internal organs, but not your eyes or skin.

**Primary physician.** Your advance health care directive will require you to identify the physician that you consider the most familiar with your overall health and state of mind. This is important, so that if there is any question as to the proper interpretation of your medical wishes, your primary care physician (rather than, say, an emergency room doctor who may never have met you before) will be called in to decide what medical actions are consistent with your advance health care directive.

## Get health care documents witnessed legally and make sure everyone involved in your care has copies or knows how to get access to copies.

After you've put what you want in writing, sign it, and be sure to have it properly witnessed and/or notarized according to the laws of your state. (If you have used a computer program to help you prepare your advance health care directive, you should search for the instructions pertaining to your state and follow them exactly.) Send copies to your primary care physician, your lawyer, your heirs, and anyone else you believe should be kept aware of your wishes regarding your medical care.

## Ask to review the hospital's *informed consent* form several days in advance of your surgery, if possible.

If you're like most patients on the way to the OR, here's how it goes with your informed consent form: About forty minutes before surgery, someone hands you a three-page, single-spaced document and tells you to read it and sign at the bottom. The pages are photocopies of photocopies so many times over that it's hard to make out many of the smudged words. Besides, it's full of medical jargon that you may not understand. But you get the gist of it: It tells you that anything can go wrong, you could end up seriously impaired, you could end up quadriplegic, you could die, and you agree that it would be nobody's fault. You can't find anything in the document that says you have any rights.

What if you don't sign it? Then no surgery. And you know you need the surgery—so of course you sign it. So you sigh and tell yourself that if the hospital botches the operation completely (meaning, they leave a sponge in you or they take out the wrong organ), surely you'll be able to find a lawyer sharp enough to poke some holes in those legalistic phrases that you signed giving up your right to sue.

Well, you'd probably be right. The hospital still has to treat you according to prevailing medical standards. No matter what the informed consent form says, they can't get away with gross negligence. So sign, and have your operation with peace of mind. As long as there are lawyers to take cases for 40 percent of any award in a malpractice case, you'll be able to bring a case.

On the other hand, if you can avoid being forced into signing anything in ignorance and haste, you'll be in a better position later on. So as soon as you know the name of the hospital where your procedure will be done, see if you can get hold of a copy of the informed consent form used for procedures like yours. Read it over at home, at your leisure. If there are phrases or clauses that you don't understand, by all means call to speak to someone in the hospital's administrative offices who can answer your questions. If you're still concerned, you might want to let your family lawyer take a look at the document. He or she can probably reassure you of rights you have that cannot be waived away, regardless of the language of the form.

**Be certain that the terms of your informed consent are broad enough to cover the full range of medical responses that you may want during your surgery.**
Doctors don't automatically have the right to treat a body part not covered by your consent form. If, in the course of surgery, your doctor discovers another area that must be treated surgically, he or she can do so only if it is an absolute medical necessity. Otherwise, the surgeon is obligated to wait until you are awake and able to consider the matter, which could mean you will have to undergo another operation at a later date. Your best way to avoid such a circumstance is to include in your informed consent form language authorizing your surgeon to effect any surgical repairs that in his or her best judgment are in order.

If you do wish to give your surgeon what is, in effect, carte blanche to operate on you, you should work through with him or her what response you want for all plausible outcomes. You must also consider the degree of confidence you have in your surgeon's judgment and his or her understanding of your desires. I particularly recommend careful consideration of this matter to patients with cancer, HIV, or other serious diseases that commonly entail interrelated surgeries.

On the lighter side, you could use your expanded consent form to get double duty out of your plastic surgeon. Let's say you've come in to have some unsightly scar tissue on your arm taken care of. As you're being prepared for minor surgery, you might ask, "Oh, by the way, while you're at it, would you mind taking off this mole on my neck?" Maybe she'll agree, and maybe she won't. (If she does, expect to be billed for it.) She may take one look at it, shrug, and say, "Sorry, your consent form doesn't cover this." But if you remind her that you amended your consent form to authorize any surgical action that seems appropriate under the circumstances, that mole will be history. If your consent form is too limited, ask if you can write in your okay for the additional work on the spot and initial the change. If your surgeon is flexible, that should be all that's needed.

**Consider under what circumstances you might wish to limit your informed consent to specific actions or set other limits on your medical care.**
On the other hand (to continue with the example directly above), you might be prudent to keep your surgeries separate, to permit each case to be considered with greater care. If you have a family history of melanoma or you are fair skinned and have not protected your skin from sun damage in the past, you are at increased risk of having a form of skin cancer. In that case, it would make sense for you to get a referral to a dermatologist to find out whether the mole is malignant and if so, to create a skin cancer treatment plan that includes far more than a simple excision of the mole.

Anesthesia provides another example of an area of medicine in which informed consent can be a complicated business. Here's an example I've often encountered in my practice: A patient comes into the hospital for shoulder surgery. I have his consent to administer general anesthesia, but there is another service I could provide that would give him tremendous relief post-operatively. I can do a nerve block of the shoulder that would deliver pain relief for hours after his operation. If there is time and the opportunity before the start of surgery, I discuss this option with him. It's my obligation to warn him of all possible complications, even those that are only remotely possible, such as hitting a blood vessel, or hitting a lung and having it collapse. Most of the time, patients agree to assume the risk to enjoy the benefits, and they amend the consent form to allow me to proceed. Some patients, for whatever reason, say no. That's their choice, and I would never dream of arguing with them or trying to second-guess their motives.

**Understand the phrase *"against medical advice,"* and consider under what circumstances you might invoke your right to refuse to follow your doctor's recommendations.**
It's your body, and if you're over eighteen and legally competent to make your own decisions, you have the absolute right to refuse any medical procedure. When a patient decides not to proceed with surgery despite a doctor's insistence that it's medically necessary, you could call it a case of "informed *lack* of consent." Under these circumstances the doctor will generally flag the patient's chart with the initials "AMA," meaning that the patient is acting against medical advice.

Patients who feel they're ready to go home sometimes sign themselves out of the hospital AMA, when doctors believe they need further treatment to regain their health or to survive. Frequently AMA choices are made on religious grounds: For example, Jehovah's Witnesses refuse to accept blood transfusions, which they believe to be forbidden by a certain passage in the Bible. The patients in these cases usually die rather than violate their religious beliefs.

**Know what constitutes malpractice and how hospitals and clinics protect themselves against hiring doctors with a history of losing malpractice cases.**
Knowing the criteria for malpractice suits before you have surgery does not mean you'll be litigious. It's "just in case" learning that equips

you with the information you need to be on the alert about your health care—knowledge that will also help you in your dealing with your insurance company and in selecting or changing doctors in the future.

According to legal experts, the following conditions must be met before you can make a malpractice claim:

- You and your doctor must have a doctor-patient relationship, that is, a relationship in which this physician had a duty to you.

- There was a breach of the duty. For example, if you hired a surgeon to remove your damaged right ovary and he removed your functioning left one instead, that would be a breach of duty. I've picked an extreme case; usually the alleged breach is not so clear-cut and the case involves some interpretation of the "standard of care" for that procedure.

- The breach of the duty caused you harm. Your doctor may have had a duty to take out your tonsils. Perhaps he noticed that your adenoids were also inflamed and removed them as well. Did that cause you harm? No, so the third criterion for a malpractice suit is not present. By removing your adenoids, however, he did leave himself open to a battery suit. Battery involves unlawful contact with your body. There would also be the issue of the surgeon's lack of specific informed consent, a separate cause of legal action against the surgeon.

There are doctors who've been sued who deserved legal trouble and there are doctors who've endured completely groundless lawsuits. The **National Practitioner Data Bank (NPDB),** which is currently closed to the lay public, maintains a record of all charges lodged against medical practitioners. Congress created the databank in 1990 to keep track of physicians who have been disciplined by medical boards or professional societies, paid on malpractice suits, and/or had hospital privileges suspended for more than 30 days. The impetus behind the law was to stop doctors from hiding a bad record simply by moving to another state or applying for a new medical license.

The rationale for keeping the NPDB restricted to other health care professionals was that the restriction is necessary to encourage physicians and hospitals to submit information voluntarily to the database. Because it's routine for insurance companies to settle many malpractice claims, whether or not malpractice was committed, many doctors are listed who have done nothing wrong. Consumers lack the resources, supposedly, to investigate cases thoroughly, but hospital administrators and others involved in hiring will know how to judge the record fairly—according to those who supported the bill.

However, much of the information found in the closed database is now available to the general public, thanks to a consumer interest organization called the Public Citizen Health Research Group, directed

---

*Annie went in for* long-overdue gall bladder surgery. It was long overdue because she had been misdiagnosed for more than a year. But Annie habitually keeps good records, a skill she puts to good use daily in her work, which involves collecting marketing and sales data for software companies. When she finally went through the procedure, she had complications because the surgeon nicked another organ—but Annie didn't know that at first. She reports, "I stayed in the hospital for days, with no one telling me exactly what was going on. They gave me so much pain medicine—that's good in the sense that I was in pain and needed it, but bad because I wasn't sure what was happening."

Annie's friends, many of whom had been in close touch with her throughout the ordeal, exchanged insights and observations through emails. After she recovered, she and her friends got together and studied the notes and observations they had made throughout her hospitalization. The written record proved that she met the three general conditions (listed on page 111) needed to prove malpractice, and she proceeded with a strong case against her surgeon.

---

by a physician, Dr. Sidney Wolfe. The nonprofit organization publishes a multi-volume directory of doctors who have been disciplined, compiled from data gathered from all the states' various medical regulatory agencies and professional boards. The directory is also available as a CD-rom. To purchase the directory for your region at a cost of twenty dollars, log onto ***www.citizen.org/hrg/qdsite/orderform.htm*** or contact the organization at 1600 20th Street, NW, Washington, DC 20009. Telephone: 202-588-1000.

In Chapter 7, "In the Hospital," you will find several tips designed to help you recognize and prevent instances of malpractice before they occur. (See the tip on page 141 about hand washing, the tip on page 150 about questioning medications, and the tips on pages 142-143 about speaking clearly about what you're in for and identifying the body part to be operated on.)

### Avoid important legal and financial decisions in the days before and after surgery.

Before surgery you're probably under a lot of stress, and you may be in considerable pain. Your mental faculties can be as worn down as your physical strength. After your surgery, anesthetic drugs may linger in your body for many hours or even a day, affecting both your mind and body. You might think you'll bounce back quickly and be as sharp as you ever were the very next day, but in my practice, I've found it's common for patients to need at least a week before their heads are clear enough to deal with complicated matters. It's difficult to judge yourself objectively when you've been on strong medications for a while. What I've seen is that patients typically regret any stock trades or other financial decisions made from a hospital bed. My advice is to let someone you trust deal with your business until you're home and you feel fully up to the job. As for those who would pressure you to get back to work before you're feeling well enough to handle it— I think they make it quite clear what sort of people they are. You have to ask yourself, "Do I want to follow the advice of someone who cares so little for my well being?"

# CHAPTER 6

# Getting Ready to Go:
# Packing and Other Practical Details

B y now you should know what hospital you'll be using, who will
be working on you, and more or less what will happen once you're
under anesthesia. You'll also have a fairly good idea of what to expect when you wake up. If you made your choices based primarily on
the track records and the confidence-inspiring manner of the people
and institutions involved, you should be in very good shape as far as
your safety is concerned.

In this chapter the focus is on the less crucial, but still important,
matter of your comfort. In even the finest hospitals with the most
diligent staff, there are disruptions and inconveniences and petty irri-
tations that can turn even the most successful medical procedure into
what seems like a prison sentence. In most cases, however, patients
can take steps to protect themselves from (or at least greatly reduce)
the discomforts of a hospital stay. The suggestions below should go a
long way toward helping you achieve that goal.

**Get a private room, if at all possible.**
This is such an important piece of advice for your comfort that I'd
say do it even if it means a putting a strain on your budget. When
you're feeling at your worst, that's when you *least* need to worry
about how to get along with a roommate.

Of course, your insurance covers only a semiprivate room; you
can expect to pay anywhere from sixty to two hundred dollars more
per day out of pocket for your own room. But think of what you save
yourself from: an unknown person, with an unknown sleeping

schedule, and unknown friends and relatives showing up to visit; with TV, radio, and music tastes that may drive you around the bend; personal habits that may gross you out; maybe snoring; or needing the lights out or needing to keep them on; a whole new set of germs and fluids and bodily wastes to be concerned about; all in addition to the inevitable parade of doctors and nurses performing necessary hospital procedures that hurt. It's bad enough to have to deal your own pain, but why throw in someone else's on top of that?

Under certain circumstances a private room will be part of standard care; for example, in cases requiring limited patient contact to prevent the spread of a highly contagious disease. Some hospitals have a policy to provide a private room for all patients after open heart surgery or for all patients undergoing treatment for what may be a terminal illness. If you fit your hospital's criteria for a mandatory private room, this is something your patient advocate should look into on your behalf.

### Get the nicest room you can.

If you toured the hospital prior to scheduling your surgery and you followed the advice in Chapter 2 about noting which rooms were the most desirable, you should definitely mention your preferences upon admission.

It may be that there's little choice in the room you end up with, but if there are different types of rooms available and the person in charge of the assignment is aware that you'd prefer one over another, you'll probably get your choice. At least there's no harm in asking.

Here are some considerations to keep in mind when considering which hospital rooms are best:

- **Location.** Is it on the sunny side of the street? (That's good if you like rays, bad if you want your room dark while you take a daytime nap.)
- **Size.** Is the room large enough to accommodate you and all the doctors, nurses, and aides who will need to examine you and administer treatments? Or is it the proverbial broomcloset, so small that two visitors will have to come in on piggyback?

- **View.** Are you looking at an ugly air shaft, or do you look out over a courtyard garden?

- **Noise.** Are you near a waiting area/lounge with a big TV that's always on, or are you near a vending machine that makes a thunking sound every time a can comes down the chute? Or are you at the quiet end of the corridor?

- **Furniture.** Do some rooms have comfortable chairs in good condition, while others have chairs that look like they've been there since World War II? Is there a bed-tray on wheels that can easily be positioned to the height that's most comfortable? Are the bed controls easily accessible and simple to operate?

- **Closets and cabinets.** Is there a place to hang your clothes and store your empty suitcase so that no one has to trip over it coming and going? Also, is there at least one storage space in the room for nurses to quickly grab extra supplies (rubber gloves, tubing, tape, etc.), or do they have to go to their supply room at the end of another corridor for any little thing they need?

- **Décor.** Is the paint or wallpaper fresh and bright, or is the room painted that dull institutional green?

- **Lighting control.** Do some rooms have blackout shades so that you can make it totally dark, or are there just flimsy venetian blinds with a few slats missing?

- **Ventilation system.** Is the room stuffy and overheated? Or is it drafty and chilly? Do patients have the ability to make it warmer or cooler, or is the thermostat setting completely out of their hands?

- **TV.** Is it mounted on a swing-arm so that you can bring it down to a comfortable viewing level while you're in bed, or is it hung up on a platform on the wall near the ceiling at the far end of the room?

- **Bathroom facilities.** Is it a straight shot from your bed to the toilet, or do you have to maneuver around tables, chairs, and medical equipment every time you need to go? (Remember, you're probably going to find it hard at first to get in and out of bed unassisted, and you might be dragging an IV pole around with you, too.)

- **Art and wall hangings.** Are there cheerful posters or paintings on the walls? Are there religious icons, statues, or other symbols that you would like to have in view, and if not, would you be allowed to bring in your own from home? For those staying in a hospital affiliated with a different faith than your own, are there symbols on the wall that you might be allowed to have put away during your stay?

### If price is no object for you, find out if your hospital has a luxury wing.

These days some hospitals are becoming more like businesses in the way they compete for customers. One of the ways to get patients to prefer one hospital over another is to offer a higher level of comfort to those who can afford the best. While the standard of medical care is the same for patients in the luxury wing as in the rest of the hospital, the number and quality of amenities is far superior, comparable with that found in a fine hotel (at least that's what the hospital's ads usually imply).

In the luxury wing you are served gourmet food cooked by chefs; you wear fine gowns and robes of Egyptian cotton, not the one-size-fits-all dishtowel that everyone else is made to wear; and the room's furnishings and draperies have been chosen by a top interior designer.

Elizabeth Taylor, when she was a patient at Washington (DC) Hospital Center, reportedly stayed in a suite redecorated especially for her. Patients coming to stay at the hospital right after she checked out were known to ask for "Elizabeth Taylor's room"—and no doubt some lucky patients would get it.

### Pack with your comfort in mind.

If you are scheduled for anything more than same-day surgery, think carefully about what to bring to the hospital. My philosophy is that it's better to have too much than to be calling friends and family with this or that request. Your brother may not know where to find your extra reading glasses or your fleece-lined slippers, so if you think you might conceivably want them, pack them. Almost everyone needs and receives help when they're packing up for their discharge and bringing their bags down to the car, so don't worry about packing more than you'll be able to carry by yourself.

The following box lists things to bring and not bring.

---

**Things that you *definitely* want to bring are:**

- Your toothbrush and your own favorite brand of toothpaste.

- Brush/comb, razor/shaving cream, and other essential toiletries.

- Eyeglasses and case (for those who wear contact lenses, see the tip on page 139).

- Paperback books and magazines (nothing too heavy to hold up in bed)—books on tape are an excellent idea.

- Personal stereo with headphones (battery-operated only— you probably won't be allowed to plug anything into hospital electric outlets).

- Instructions from your surgeon or other doctors that you need to follow while you are in the hospital.

- Test results (such as the film from your last MRI) that you are expected to hand-deliver to your surgeon before your procedure begins.

- List of your medications or a placard with any medical notes (such as warning of a drug allergy) you want to be sure no one will miss.

- Personal phone book or personal digital assistant with names and contact information for anyone you need to be able to reach during your hospital stay (especially numbers for all your doctors, including their home numbers, if you can get them).

- Special devices or accessories for your special needs (for example, a special seat cushion for hemorrhoid sufferers, hearing aids for the hearing impaired, orthodontic

---

appliances—but see the caution on page 139 about removing all appliances before surgery).

**Things you *may* want to bring are:**

- Your preferred brand of soap and shampoo.
- Skin moisturizer (but don't apply it before surgery).
- Your own pajamas/nightgown and robe (but not anything you'd hate to see ruined by bleeding, spills, or stains). Take note of what body part will be affected by your procedure and avoid anything tight-fitting in that area. Choose sleepwear that opens easily to allow staff to examine you, administer medications, and monitor your body functions as is necessary for your treatment.
- Your own pillow(s) and/or special cushions. First check with the hospital and doctor to be sure there's no rule or medical reason against using your own pillow.
- Eyeshades.
- Earplugs or a small tabletop white noise machine (battery only).
- Hand-held electronic game player and cartridges (such as the Gameboy)
- Deck of cards, puzzle books, other pen-and-paper games you can play solo or with a visitor.

**Things you definitely should *not* bring are:**

- Jewelry.
- Money/wallet (hospitals have too many strangers wandering around and things do get stolen).
- Perfume or other heavily scented personal care products (which may mask smells that warn of various medical problems).
- Cigarettes (there's not a hospital in the country that isn't a smoke-free zone).
- Alcoholic beverages (will almost certainly be banned because alcohol interacts with so many drugs).

**Bring your list of the medications you currently take.**

In Chapter 3, I discussed the necessity of making sure your doctor is aware of all medications you take (prescription and non-prescription, including vitamins and other supplements). It's even more important to make sure that hospital staff members know what medications and supplements you're on. Of course, they'll be getting orders from doctors about what to give you, but orders can (and all too often do) get confused. It's a safeguard for you to have your own list with you. That way if there is any discrepancy between what the nurse says you are to take and what your doctor has told you to take, you can say, "Wait a minute. We need to check this out first." This is such an important safety tip that I repeat it in Chapter 7, "In the Hospital," and again in Chapter 9, "When You Have No Time to Plan." The later tips include suggestions for the format of the list and keeping it someplace handy, so that you can just grab it when you need to go to the hospital in a hurry.

**Make sure you have all your contact information (including all your doctors' office and emergency telephone numbers), admission forms, insurance approvals, test results, and any other paperwork you are supposed to bring in.**

Here's what you *don't* want to happen: You're all packed up, you're emotionally psyched, you're at the admitting desk, and you're ready to have the procedure—but it's not going to happen, all because you don't have that one little piece of paper that must be in your doctor's hands (or your insurer's hands, or the hospital clerk's hands) before things can proceed. So be absolutely clear that you know all the paperwork and documents that you are responsible for bringing with you on the date of your procedure, and make sure nothing gets left at home. The tip below will help you accomplish this.

**Create a packing checklist and check off each item as you put it in your bag.**

This is the method pilots use before each flight to make sure they have everything (because you don't want to get up to 7,000 feet and discover you're missing the one navigational chart that will get you to your destination). The story in the box below shows why this is such a handy idea.

***Jay was scheduled*** for a lumbar laminectomy, a procedure to cut out tissue from herniated disks in the vertebrae. To perform the operation, the surgeon needs to have on hand the MRI film showing which specific disk had ruptured. That film was kept at the MRI center where the test had been done. The surgeon told Jay to make arrangements to pick up the film ahead of time and bring it in with him on the morning of the procedure. Jay knew that there could be no operation without the film. So he put the envelope containing the film right by the front door, where he would be sure to see it on his way out. He also put sticky notes saying "<u>REMEMBER FILM</u>" on the desk in the front hall and on the door. The morning of the surgery, his alarm went off at 4:00 A.M. and he got up and started to get ready to go. He and his wife knew they needed to be at the admitting desk of the hospital by 5:30 A.M. They showered, dressed, grabbed his overnight bag, and were in the car and on the road to the hospital by 4:30, both feeling great that they were ahead of schedule. It wasn't until they were almost at the hospital that they realized they'd left the film behind. Somehow in the pre-dawn darkness, with all their rushing around and their nervousness over the procedure to come, they'd managed to overlook all the sticky notes and reminders as well as the envelope itself near the front door.

Fortunately, they arrived so early that Jay's wife had time to turn around and drive home, retrieve the film, and return to the hospital before the surgeon had arrived. Things went off without another hitch, but they did learn an important lesson: *Don't leave for the hospital without having checked that you have with you every item deemed necessary for the surgery to proceed.*

**Put your name and telephone number on all your things.**
You should have a clear, visible luggage tag on your suitcase and some identifying information on everything you've packed in it. The easiest way to mark your things is to use a fine-point, indelible-ink marker (a laundry marker works well) to write your name and phone number on each item you're bringing along. That includes books and magazines, unless you intend to leave them behind for anyone who might want them after you're done with them.

**Find out where your things will be stored or who will keep hold of them during surgery.**
You probably won't know your room assignment until your surgery is over. Whoever accompanies you to the hospital should be the one left in charge of your things. That person can find out if there is a safe storage area, or can simply hold onto your things until you're moved to your hospital room. If you're on your own, ask a nurse or a hospital volunteer to help you out with this simple task, but only after you've first made sure that your helper's shift goes at least until the time you're released from the recovery room.

**Pack a separate totebag or backpack with the things you need on the day of surgery.**
Your packed suitcase and the bag with the clothes you wore to the hospital will be put aside for you until you have a room, but you can and should set aside some things in a separate bag that you'll be glad you kept with you while you are waiting and getting ready for your procedure.

Even if your procedure is set for first thing in the morning, in all likelihood you will still do lots of waiting around. Emergencies crop up that can delay things by hours, but even without emergencies, delays are an inevitable fact of hospital life: Rooms need to prepared, staff members may be late getting in, medical equipment must to be moved into place, test results get lost—these are just a few of the dozens of reasons for delay. The wait won't be so annoying if you come prepared. In your totebag or backpack you should stash a good book (or maybe a selection of magazines), your personal tape or CD player with the kind of music you think you'd find soothing or enjoyable while you wait, and maybe a book on tape. Hand-held electronic games can also be a great distraction. If you've studied yoga, meditation, or any other stress-relieving technique, then by all means bring along whatever easily portable aids you employ in your exercises.

If you're going in for an outpatient procedure, you'll probably be given a locker for your bag while you're in surgery. If you'll be admitted for overnight or longer, make sure that someone is assigned to keep tabs on this bag during your procedure and make sure it's delivered to your hospital room as soon as the room assignment has been made.

**Find out if you can plug your portable radio, TV, or computer into the hospital's electrical system; if not, bring batteries.**
Many hospitals won't allow you to plug "foreign" devices into their electrical systems. You might also find that bringing your radio, television, or cellular phone into the hospital room is pointless because the reception is so bad. The best thing to do if you want to bring any type of equipment into the room is to ask in advance. You certainly don't want to lug your own portable TV to the hospital if it turns out that every room has a TV mounted on a swing-arm for easy viewing and operation by push-buttons built into the bed frame.

**If you will be in the hospital for a long time, find out if you can have a VCR.**
TV is fine for a few days, but if you will be in for much longer than that, you will probably want alternatives to the usually limited channel selection found on most hospital cable TV systems. Some hospitals will hook up a VCR for any patient who is in for a long stay; others will allow you to make arrangements to have a VCR hooked up; still others say "no" to use of anything electronic except what they already provide for you.

If you do get turned down, I would urge you to appeal to the directors of the hospital. I think it's been proven that patients do better by far when they're entertained than when they're bored—as studies have shown (see next tip).

**Watch comedy videos to help you recuperate.**

A 1999 study involving heart attack patients showed that the half who watched humorous videos regularly after their attack had significantly lower rates of recurrence. That's an amazing result! I think it's also fair to assume that humor aids in the recovery of other types of hospital patients, too.

Believing in the old saying that "laughter is the best medicine," the Hebrew Home of Greater Washington has a program called "Ha!ha!logy," directed by Jackie Kwan, which provides light entertainment to their patients and to those in area hospitals as well.

Your hospital probably does not have such a service, but there should be nothing preventing you from starting your own self-service unit. If you'll be in the hospital for more than a few days, look into arrangements for getting a VCR hooked up in your rooom, and then pack up the funniest movies you can buy or rent. Know your own taste in humor, though. You'll probably want to avoid seeing any "black humor" classics, like *Harold and Maude* (it's all jokes about death) or physically graphic humor, like *Osmosis Jones,* in which Bill Murray plays a patient whose insides (shown in lifelike computer-generated animation) are surgically explored for maximum gross-out value. I would also suggest you avoid any blood-chilling horror movies or thrillers that can really set your heart racing.

If it turns out to be impossible to get a VCR, remember that books and audio-tapes can be funny, too.

**After same day surgery, make sure that a responsible person will take you home and will take care of you at home if you need it.**

On the day of surgery I've sometimes had to cancel cases because the patient did not make arrangements for a responsible person to take him or her home.

If you're set to have anything except the most limited form of local anesthesia, you *must* follow this advice. A cab won't do, either. You can't expect a cab driver to walk you upstairs, get you an ice pack, tuck you in bed, or make you a cup of tea to sip after checking to see that you've taken the right dose of your pain medication.

Even for those who aren't expecting to need any form of anesthesia, who are legally permitted to drive themselves home, I still strongly recommend bringing along a friend to help at discharge time. You can't be sure how you'll react to the procedure. There could be complications, and you may end up having drugs you didn't know you'd need. You may feel faint or nauseated, when you were sure you'd be just fine, or you just may feel a tiny bit shaky on your feet. In all cases you'll be better off leaving the driving to someone else. The two examples in the box on page 127 illustrate the point.

**Even if you're having an outpatient procedure, pack for an overnight stay, just in case.**
Even the simplest procedures can become complicated. In this imperfect universe there is simply no way to guarantee yourself a perfect outcome, so the best you can do is prepare yourself to deal with the unexpected. You never want your child to be stuck in daycare, wondering where you are. You don't even want your car housed in a high-priced lot overnight if you can avoid it. What you need to do is to think through carefully all your obligations and figure out how they could be met in some alternative manner if you ended up staying in the hospital longer than planned. Tell everyone who might possibly need to know about your coming trip to the hospital. Make sure each person understands what he or she is supposed to do if they don't hear from you or your patient advocate by a certain time of day.

Part of your preparation should include bringing anything with you that you would need if you had to stay overnight (for example, your toothbrush and toothpaste, a change of underwear, any medications you need to take at night or the following day).

**If you'll be awake during your procedure, find out whether you can use your portable CD or tape player to keep you distracted while it's going on.**
More and more procedures are being done with patients lightly sedated or completely awake. Anything done under local anesthesia or with a nerve block, such as a knee arthroscopy, fits this bill. If your surgeon doesn't mind, you might like to pass the time while she's working on

**Robin went in for** a dilation and curettage (D&C) of her uterus following a miscarriage of a much-wanted pregnancy. Her gynecologist told her it was a routine procedure and that she'd be able to go home an hour or so after the D&C was complete. It was true, she was up and walking around within an hour, but she certainly didn't feel normal. She felt weepy and depressed, although she didn't want to tell her doctor, or even her husband, how low she was feeling. Good thing she had arranged to have her husband drive her home. On the way home, Robin completely fell apart. First, she was overcome by waves of nausea, which came on her so quickly she did not even have time to roll the car window all the way down and lean out. Then, soiled and miserable, she fell into a crying jag that lasted the rest of the drive. She was just thankful she had her husband with her to bring her upstairs, get her to bed, and take care of their three-year-old daughter, so that she could sleep the rest of day and into the night. She awoke the next morning feeling a great deal better.

*********

**Jane had claustrophobia,** triggered by having been in the confines of the MRI machine. After the test she felt so shaky that she couldn't drive for an hour. Being in a closed and noisy space for twenty-five minutes, unable to move any body part, was torture to her. Here's what she learned from the experience: "I recommend that anytime people go in for a procedure they've never had before that someone be outside waiting. I don't care if it's getting a tooth pulled—if you've never had it done before, you don't know how you're going to react to the medicine or the procedure."

you by listening to music, a relaxation tape, a book on tape, or anything that you think would help take your mind off the procedure (especially if there is any drilling or other noise associated with it).

> **Rosemary had her psychologist** create a tape specifically for her, so that throughout her knee surgery, she would hear key words and stories that triggered good feelings. Her psychologist also recorded a follow-up tape focused on recovery and therapy that Rosemary used in the days after the surgery.

### Find out how the food is at the hospital.

You've heard about hospital food, of course. In some hospitals it even makes airline food look good by comparison. It's a smart idea to get some advance notice about the quality of food where you'll be going. Do you know anyone who was a patient at the same hospital within the last year or so? If so, ask them how the food was. If the answer comes back, "inedible" or "made me feel sicker than I already was," then go on to the tip below.

### Find out whether there are alternatives to using the hospital's food service.

Ask a hospital administrator if someone can bring you sandwiches from home or maybe pick up a prepared meal from a deli or carry-out restaurant. You might be able to phone for pizza or Chinese food delivery. Of course, you should check first with your doctor to find out if you're under any dietary restrictions for medical reasons, and if so, for how long.

For those who will be eating the hospital's food, it's still a good idea to ask about the rules for outside food being brought in. Can a visitor bring you a home-baked pie? You don't want someone to put a lot of effort into pleasing you with a favorite dish, only to find out that you can't even have a bite.

### Find out how your special dietary needs will be met.

First, make sure your dietary restrictions are known. For example, if you are diabetic, make sure the hospital staff is aware that you can't have anything high in sugar or fats, or if you have high cholesterol, let them know that you follow a high-fiber, low-fat diet. Also, make sure you have mentioned any religious or cultural dietary practices that are important to you: For example, you may keep Kosher, observe Halal food preparation rules, or follow the Mormon practice of avoiding anything that contains caffeine, or you may be a vegan (someone who avoid all foods made with animal products, including dairy products). The larger the hospital, the greater the likelihood that the catering service will be able to accommodate your special needs.

If you learn that the hospital cannot supply you with the sort of meals you require, then follow the advice above about checking to see if you can have food brought in from the outside. If the answer is yes, be clear on when you are first allowed to have solid food after your procedure, and what medical restrictions, if any, must be followed. Also make sure the person delivering the food knows about safe food handling and transport.

### Find out what the visiting policy is at the hospital.

Hospitals vary greatly in their visiting policies. Some will let only one person in at a time; some will permit an entire family to visit. You may have to authorize your visitors in advance. If so, the time to deal with the matter is now, while you still are up and alert, and have time to give some thought to the matter. Do you want your children to be able to see you? (Consider how you might look to them with tubes and drains coming out of your bandaged body. Will they be scared?) Do you want friends or other family members to be allowed to bring their children? It's not only a matter of knowing the hospital rules, you also need to make your potential visitors aware of your wishes.

### If the visiting policy doesn't suit you, find out if rules can be bent.

You need to find out how flexible the hospital is about its visiting rules before you're set to go. The worst thing would be to have your beloved but former in-laws come all the way across the country to see you during your recovery from cancer surgery only to learn that they aren't permitted in because they don't fit the hospital definition of "family members."

At the request of a doctor or therapist, however, rules can often be changed to suit the patient's needs. For example, if the physical therapist wants to demonstrate how family members can assist the patient in performing special exercises, she may request that all key people be allowed in the patient's room at once. If you lack such an explicit medical reason to change the rules, you can always make the case that having loved ones around you is important for your emotional well-being and an essential part of your recovery.

### Find out if the hospital will protect you against unwanted visitors.

In addition to being sure the hospital will allow in those whom you wish to see, you want to be assured that they will keep out those you would rather not see. If it's going to stress you out to see your boss while you're laid up and unable to get anything done on that project you know is overdue, you don't want to have to explain that to him. Find out if the hospital staff will shield you from unwanted drop-ins. This is a question to raise with the hospital administrative staff in advance of your stay. If the answer turns out to be that it's up to you to tell unwanted visitors to stay away, then make sure you have a patient advocate who will act as your effective gatekeeper.

### If you're a light sleeper, look for ways to get a good night's sleep in the hospital.

Hospitals are up and running twenty-four hours a day, which means there's light and sound all around the clock. The doors to patients' rooms are usually left open to allow nurses and other staff members to look in whenever they like. The floors are uncarpeted and things clatter when they drop. Other patients turn the TV volume way up. People are always coming in to do things to you. And yet they continually urge you to "get some rest."

If you're a light sleeper, it's hard to know how. Maybe you will be put on drugs that will put you out for a few hours between blood-sticks. If you're not, I suggest you use eyeshades, ear plugs, and possibly a white noise machine (a battery-operated tabletop appliance that produces a whooshing or whirring sound designed to mask other, more irritating sounds).

You should also try asking that staff members who must interrupt your sleep to take vital signs or administer medications combine their visits into the minimum number possible. Why should the nurse who comes to check on your blood pressure be followed fifteen minutes later—just as you've managed to doze off again—by a group of medical students making rounds? Why can't the person who comes to remove your meal tray wait until you've finished your nap? Certainly you should make these very reasonable requests and complain to hospital administrators if the interruptions to your sleep go on as before.

### Don't overeat in the evening before your surgery.

You heard your doctor warn, "Nothing to eat or drink after midnight on the night before your surgery!" That doesn't mean you can go to your favorite all-you-can-eat smorgasbord and pig out until 11:45 P.M. Sure, you're in compliance with your doctor's orders, technically speaking, but you'll regret it all the same. As you lie down to sleep that night, you may feel bloated and uncomfortable. Maybe you'll have a harder time falling asleep and the next morning will feel miserable. So your safest, most sensible course is to eat a light, healthy meal at your normal dinnertime the day before. I've generally found that my surgical patients do better when their digestive tracts are relatively empty, and so I also recommend avoiding red meat, anything with a heavy cream sauce, rich desserts, and other foods that take a long time to be processed through your system.

### Don't drink alcohol the night before surgery.

Alcohol stimulates stomach acid secretion, and aspirating that during surgery spells trouble. At the very least, after an evening of drinking, you will wake up dehydrated, and may even have a hangover. Add that to the stress of surgery and the effects of anesthesia, and you'll think you've died and gone to hell.

I hope it goes without saying that you can't have any alcohol on the day of surgery, either. I've actually had patients—closet alcoholics—show up on the day of surgery with alcohol on their breath. There's nothing I can do but send them home. It's too dangerous to administer anesthesia to someone already under the influence of a powerful drug like alcohol. The real trouble comes when a person has been drinking but lies and attempts to cover it up. Anesthesiologists are trained to err on the side of caution and will refuse to provide anesthesia drugs to a patient who appears at risk for an alcohol-anesthesia drug interaction.

### If your surgery isn't set for first thing in the morning, find out if you can bend the "nothing after midnight" rule.

It's not hard to stick to the "nothing after midnight" rule when your surgery is set for first thing the next morning. It's much tougher if you're going to have to last all morning, and maybe half the afternoon as well, without food or drink. But that may not be necessary. Under newly developed guidelines on pre-operative fasting, doctors are allowing some flexibility in what they tell patients about drinking, if not eating. The focus of key studies has specifically been on the differences, especially in gastric volume and acidity, seen in patients allowed to drink clear liquids (meaning, water or clear fruit juice) until two to four hours before surgery, and the volumes seen in patients who abstained from clear liquids for more than four hours. The subjects still fasted from food, but the variable tested was whether or not results were just as good in patients allowed to drink something beforehand. The preliminary conclusion seems to be that drinking clear liquids on the same day of surgery (up to two hours beforehand) made little if any difference. But always check with the anesthesiologist at your facility about eating and drinking rules.

### To avoid having nice underwear ruined, don't wear it to the hospital.

Your doctor may tell you that you have an option of keeping on your underwear for surgery and while lying in your hospital bed. That's fine, but be sure you're not wearing anything you really care to keep. Many circumstances during surgery can lead to ruined underwear. For example, in administering an epidural anesthetic, the doctor or nurse will swab your back with a solution like Betadine, a rust-colored iodine disinfectant. It will probably run down your backside and color whatever it touches with a stain that no laundry product could possibly remove.

### Do not shave yourself in preparation for surgery.

A lot of people will come into the surgical area and say, "Look, doc, I've already shaved for you!" Don't do that unless shaving that part of your body is routine for you, because you just might cut yourself, which will leave you open to infection. Let the surgical staff do it for you—it's their job, after all.

### If you occasionally have trouble sleeping, ask for a sedative for the night before surgery.

You really need a good night's sleep before surgery. Ask your doctor for a sleeping pill if you think that anxiety or pain will interfere in any way with your rest.

### If you smoke, avoid doing so for at least a few days before surgery.

Smokers, if ever you needed a reason to quit for good, you've found it the minute you learn you're going to need surgery. But if you've tried and tried, and just haven't managed to give the stuff up, at least give your lungs a break from the intake of toxic smoke in the days just prior to surgery. While you're in the operating room under general anesthesia, you'll need every breathing advantage you can possibly get—for both your comfort and your safety. Smoking depresses the action of cilia, hair-like sweepers in your wind passages. Stopping

*Barbara, a 67-year-old woman* who broke her femur, kicked her lifelong smoking habit in the hospital. She attributes her success to the complete schedule change as well as the compelling distraction of her broken leg. Barbara says, "This may sound weird, but I think that breaking my leg may have saved my life. I feel so much younger and more energetic now that I can breathe."

smoking just a few days before surgery has been shown to improve your ciliary function, that is, it improves your ability to clear phlegm and secretions from your lungs. Staying smoke free right after surgery will also help your healing process. Among other things, smoking robs your body of oxygen and vitamin C, both of which your body needs to heal.

Consult your doctor about any pharmacological approach you're considering using to quit smoking, though. This would include nicotine patches and gum. They are delivery systems for the stimulant drug nicotine, and you need to be sure your doctor is informed about any such use, just as you informed your doctor about all other medications you use.

### If you have asthma, bring your inhaler with you to the hospital, and ask your doctor if your condition warrants a pre-surgical breathing treatment.

As an asthma sufferer, you probably know the various environments and circumstances that can trigger an attack. For many people, stress is a distinct cause. Anticipate that the stress of surgery could bring on the symptoms, so be prepared with your inhaler. This may save you the expense of more costly respiratory treatments should you start wheezing right before surgery.

Some doctors will have patients with severe asthma take a breathing treatment, administered by a respiratory therapist. You will breathe humidified medicine through a mouthpiece to make you more comfortable during surgery. Yes, the treatment is more expensive than relying solely on your inhaler. For starters, you involve another department—the respiratory therapy department—in your care. Then you have the added cost of the drug delivery system and monitors that go with your special respiratory therapy. However, for those who have ever experienced a potentially life-threatening asthma attack, the expense will be more than justified by the in-surgery respiratory distress you will avoid.

### If you have a hiatal hernia or an ulcer, or if you experience frequent heartburn, ask your doctor about taking a

**nonparticulate antacid, such as** *sodium citrate,* **before surgery. If so, find out if you should bring your own supply.**
Sodium citrate is a salty-tart liquid—like salty Tang—that neutralizes stomach acid. The usual pre-surgery dosage is about 30 cc's and it's called "non-particulate" because it's a smooth liquid that contains no solid particles. Sodium citrate is an inexpensive, over-the-counter therapy, which used to be given routinely before cesarean sections (C-sections), because pregnancy makes women prone to aspirating acid into their lungs under anesthesia.

In many hospitals, it's been replaced by other, pricier acid blockers such as Tagamet (cimetidine) or Prilosec (omeprazole). If you have fit any of the following categories—you have gastro-esophogeal reflux disease (GERD), a hiatal hernia, an ulcer, or chronic heartburn— you'll probably find one of these new medicines even more effective than sodium citrate. The newer acid-blockers can reduce the damaging effects of aspiration of stomach contents into the lungs, preventing lung damage and perhaps even saving your life.

Don't take the sodium citrate without your doctor's knowledge in an attempt to save money, though. Make sure your doctor knows about your condition and has decided which approach you should follow. *Do not break the "nothing after midnight rule" by taking sodium citrate unless your doctor specifically directs you to do so.*

**If you are experiencing a flare-up of a chronic condition, delay going to the hospital, if possible, until you are stable.**
I've already mentioned some concerns of relevance to patients with asthma, GERD, hiatal hernia, and ulcers. If you fit into any of these categories, or if you have diabetes, heart disease, or any other systemic or chronic illness or condition, you want to make sure your symptoms are under good control before you subject yourself to the stress of surgery for some unrelated problem. That is to say, an asthma sufferer should not be having surgery when experiencing daily wheezing attacks; the diabetic should know how to keep his or her blood sugar within permitted limits, and the hypertension patient should be on an effective medication regime to prevent swings of blood pressure, either high or low.

If you're not sure whether you meet the criteria to have elective surgery, it's always wise to check with your primary care doctor or the specialist who treats your particular chronic condition. It isn't the surgeon's job to do a battery of tests on you to ensure that you're in shape for an operation. Of course, if the surgery is so urgently needed that it cannot be postponed long enough to allow your symptoms to be controlled, then be sure your surgeon is kept up to date on your condition and is in touch with your specialist. Together they should be able to work out a plan to deal with any complications that your condition might cause.

**Get your doctor's home telephone number.**
Some doctors will give it out, trusting their patients to call only when they really, *really* need to. They know that even in the best hospitals there can be times when the patient is being told one thing by the night resident and another thing by the head nurse. Only the doctor can clear the matter up. After-hours answering services are sometimes good at knowing when the doctor needs to respond quickly— but sometimes they're not. It's a great comfort to patients to know they can call their doctor at home directly—so if you're not offered the home number, ask.

Many doctors, of course, are unwilling to give it out (or have stopped giving it out, because too many patients called about trivial matters), and if that's the reaction you get from your doctor, be sure you have his or her after-hours number or emergency number written down in several places, and that you keep the numbers accessible while you're in the hospital.

# CHAPTER 7

# In the Hospital

Now we're down to the nitty-gritty: What actually goes on once you're admitted to the hospital, and what you can do to make sure that what's happening is just what you need and expect. Surprises in the hospital are almost always bad. Isn't the word "Oops" the most dreaded of all the things you can hear coming from a surgeon's mouth? It's not much better coming from a hospital nurse or technician, either! The idea behind the tips and suggestions in this chapter is to do everything you can to ensure that you never hear that word.

**Don't use skin cream or lotion before you come into the hospital for surgery.**

As dry as your hands and other body parts may feel, don't use skin cream before your surgery. Bathe or shower, dry off, and leave it at that. No part of your body that's recently been treated with lotion will allow surgical tape to stick to your skin. If the tape isn't sticking well, the nurses will be putting on tape and pulling it off and then retaping and pressing harder to get the tape to stick, which will be frustrating for them and uncomfortable for you. There may be difficulty setting up your IV and getting it to stay in place if the tape isn't holding as it should.

**Don't wear makeup to the hospital.**

You can't have your lipstick or foundation rubbing off on any of the tubes that will be going down your mouth and/or nose. You don't want anyone on your surgical team to get anything on their gloves that may then come into contact with the inside of your body. Worst of all would be contamination with some flaky, hard-to-remove substance like waterproof mascara. Even if your procedure will involve only local anesthetics on a remote body part (let's say it's a bunion on your foot), you still want to leave the makeup off that day, just in case you react to something and need oxygen quickly. There's never time to stop and remove makeup when something has gone wrong.

### Don't wear nail polish, false nails, or nail tips on the day of surgery.

To monitor your pulse and measure the amount of oxygen in your blood, the surgical staff uses a pulse-oximeter, which usually clips onto your finger or toe. Some clip onto your earlobe or the bridge of your nose, but they are less common. If you are wearing opaque nail polish, the pulse-oximeter cannot give a reliable reading, and the team relies on a good reading to make the appropriate judgments about your needs during surgery. To be safe, at least have one finger that has no polish of any kind on it.

### Don't wear any jewelry to surgery—and remember that this includes your wedding ring.

The primary problems with jewelry are constriction and burning. First, your extremities can swell during surgery. You don't want to put your surgeon in the position of having to remove your wedding ring with a metal cutter to avoid amputating your finger. Second, your doctor may use an electrocautery device (also called a Bovie) to seal your blood vessels and stop bleeding. Metal jewelry can conduct the electricity and lead to a nasty burn. You also don't want to have to remove your jewelry in the hospital and then wonder if it's being kept safe, especially when the solution is so simple: Take it off before you go and leave it in a safe place at home.

### Remove any and all body-piercing studs and rings before surgery.

These are jewelry, too, even though you may think of your tongue stud or the tiny rings in your genitals as permanent additions to your body. They've become so popular lately, I always make a point to check for them in my patients and make sure they're all out before I start my work. I really upset a young woman one day when I had to cut off her gold navel ring, which seemed cemented into the hole. I had a hard time getting her to understand that she was not going to be allowed to have the surgery she needed unless she let me take it out.

**Take out your contact lenses, but do bring your glasses and a case to put them in, and pack an extra pair in your suitcase.**
Regardless of the type of contact lenses you use, leave them out on the day of surgery. Your eyes can become dry and the lenses would then stick to your corneas and cause you intense pain. I'd recommend wearing your glasses to the hospital rather than taking the contacts out right before the procedure starts. It's just possible that both you and your surgical team would forget about removing the contacts ahead of time, especially when there are so many other details that need to be checked.

Of course, you'll want to see what's going on around you as much as possible after surgery, so ask a surgical nurse to tape your glasses to your chart. That way you can get them as soon as you wake up.

**Remove dentures before you go into the operating room.**
I know most patients don't like to do this, but it's really necessary. Any artificial teeth, whether full or partial dentures or just removable bridges, can chip or cause problems with intubation—you could even swallow them. Very early in my career, I was working in a hospital in Miami. A non-English-speaking lady came in, and I asked her in my best Spanish if she had any false teeth, medical appliances, or anything else on or in her body that was removable. Either she misunderstood the question or I misunderstood her answer. As we began to anesthetize her, I put the scope in to intubate her and her whole upper mouth cracked like a crab shell. I thought I had broken her head open. It was her denture plate—it sure scared the hell out of me! But I certainly found out what can happen when doctors don't have the right information on this question. (By the way, we replaced her upper plate at no cost to her.)

## If you're prone to queasiness or nausea, use a ReliefBand before surgery.

As an anesthesiologist, I'm participating in a study about the effectiveness of this FDA-approved device that you wear around your wrist. It delivers a tiny electrical charge that stimulates your body to produce anti-nausea chemicals naturally. I'm so enthusiastic about the way the product works that I strongly encourage all surgical patients to try it. There's virtually no downside to using ReliefBand; its only reported side effect is a slight tingling feeling in the fingertips, which indicates that it's working. The alternative to the ReliefBand is to use anti-nausea drugs. However, during and after surgery you're on so many other drugs that anything you can do to reduce their number is bound to be worthwhile.

See Chapter 4, "All About Anesthesia," page 87, for information on how to obtain a ReliefBand or visit the manufacturer's website at *www.reliefband.com*.

## Ask for warm blankets before surgery.

People are cold and scared when they come into the operating room, which is deliberately kept on the chilly side to restrict bacterial growth. Warmth relaxes the body (blood pressure actually drops), adds a sense of security, and dilates the veins, making for easier IV starts.

Blankets are stored in a heater in the immediate area, so the request for one or two shouldn't inconvenience anyone. In fact, those of us who work on the surgical staff enjoying draping warm blankets on patients because we become heroes. All of a sudden, patients trust us more.

Warm blankets contribute to your medical needs as much as your comfort. Chilly patients have more blood pressure problems and arrhythmias, and tend to need longer recovery times. Medical supply companies have also started to manufacture sophisticated, heated air mattresses for patients undergoing extended procedures. For these patients, the operating room team may also use heated intravenous solutions.

When you had your pre-anesthesia interview, you would have been informed if you were a candidate for these extra operating room amenities. If not, go ahead and ask for them. You may not be able to get a warmed IV circuit or a heated air mattress on short notice, but you should have no trouble getting the warmed blankets.

**If you find the operating room table too hard, ask for cushions.**
Many patients, especially those with back problems, find the operating room table uncomfortable. The tables are board-like, usually with very little cushioning—a fact that becomes clearer the longer you find yourself waiting for the anesthesia to begin. Then there are those patients whose procedures are done under a local anesthetic, who will have full sensation during the entire time they're lying down on that hard, flat metal surface. Relief may appear in the form of a cushion or small pillow, if you will only ask a nurse to provide it. The surgical team members are undoubtedly familiar with this problem and have worked out ways to provide some neck, head, knee, or back support to patients who request it.

I wouldn't suggest bringing your own pillow or foam back supporter from home, however. Given the sterility requirements of the operating room, there's little chance you'd be allowed to keep it with you. On the other hand, if you packed one in your suitcase, you stand a good shot of being able to use it later on in your own hospital room during your recovery.

**If you are especially anxious or nervous about your impending surgery, make sure your surgeon knows how you're feeling.**
Doctors don't want to see patients get worked up into a frenzy before surgery when a low dose of Valium or some other sedative that won't interfere with the planned anesthesia is all that's needed to induce a feeling of calm. Just make sure that your surgeon is aware that you could use this extra pre-surgical relief.

**If your pain reliever seems to be wearing off before a procedure, ask for more.**
Sometimes there's a delay between when you're given local anesthesia and when the procedure—suturing, for example—actually occurs. If

you feel less numb than you think you should, be sure to tell the doctor before the procedure gets started. Certainly if you're feeling pain, all you need to do is tell the surgeon what you're feeling.

**Put an ink mark on the limb or body part to be operated on.**
You've probably seen the shocking headlines about the doctor who amputated a healthy leg or the surgeon who took out a patient's functioning kidney. Probably the most frightening stories are about the rare cases in which the surgeon is a repeat offender. There was a doctor in Florida who cut the wrong foot off a patient and then within three years returned to the operating room to perform a risky operation on the wrong patient altogether.

Once you're unconscious, there is nothing you can do, but there is a simple and effective preventive measure you can take to protect yourself while you are still awake. Use a little ink on yourself to mark the body part that needs the work. You can write "This one!" or "Yes!"— and just to make sure there is no mistake, also mark the matching body part that's fine: "No! Not this one!" or "No! The other one!"

Your doctor and the nurses may have chuckle at your extreme sense of caution, but don't let that bother you. Far better for them to smile indulgently for a minute of two than to leave you with a mistake you'll have to live with for the rest of your life.

**Don't say "right" to a doctor or nurse when you mean "correct."**
Here's a story to illustrate the reason for this advice:

Barry went in for a left anterior cruciate ligament (ACL) repair. Before he went to meet the anesthesiologist, the nurse asked him a series of routine questions. She asked, "It's your left knee, right?"

Barry said, "Right."

You can guess what happened when the next person on the surgical team got the chart: "It's the right knee, I see."

"No!" Barry burst out in horror. "It's the left!"

Don't run the risk of having an Abbott and Costello "Who's on First" sort of language routine affect the outcome of your surgery. Also, keep in mind that even medical people can get their right and left mixed up. It has nothing to do with intelligence; when people are exhausted or overworked (common among hospital workers), they can make foolish errors. Now consider the normal list of surgeries for the day—right carpal tunnel, left carpal tunnel, left elbow, left knee, right knee—and you can start to see how one wrong word can put you in serious trouble.

In some hospitals, it is part of the official policy that surgeons put their initials on the correct side in ink. Everyone on the surgical team sees it and can double-check for accuracy. It's a good policy, and I'd recommend that during your pre-surgical interview, you ask whether your surgeon and your hospital follow it.

### Tell the nurses and technicians in the OR if you need them to use paper tape.

Older patients may have frail and thin skin. A common danger for them is that their skin can tear like tissue paper when silk tape is removed. People who have sensitive skin or suffer from skin diseases such as eczema or psoriasis should also be concerned about damage from regular surgical tape. Paper tape will be less irritating. If you fit any of these categories, make your request to the operating room staff before your IV is taped into place. (If you put in the request for paper tape during your pre-surgical interview, as suggested in Chapter 3, then check to see that the right type of tape is among the supplies on hand.)

### To minimize repetition, ask to have students and interns present when giving your history.

This advice is aimed mainly at patients who have been told they have a "textbook" case, that is, a case in which the symptoms lead to only one diagnosis, which in turn leads to one single and effective course of treatment. In all other cases, you will probably benefit from re-peating your history to each student, intern, resident, or attending physician who comes to see you. If there is anything at all unusual about your case, it's helpful to have many minds considering it, many pairs of eyes watching out for discrepancies in your record, and many pairs of ears listening to the details that you relate on separate occa-sions. However, in simple cases, there's no such benefit that outweighs the very real annoyance of being poked and questioned and awakened at odd hours by each new examiner in turn. When you need the rest, and you *don't* need the continuing investigation, ask the doctor in charge of your case to help you out. He or she should be able to keep control over the parade of medical caregivers who come to see you.

### Be on the lookout for doctors and nurses washing their hands. If you don't see them do it, express your concern.

You don't want to confront or insult your doctor and nurses right before surgery, but you do want to find some way to make sure that they wash their hands, even if they are putting on gloves. According to the Centers for Disease Control and Prevention, nearly 1.8 million people picked up infections in the hospital in 1999, and about 20,000 of them died from those infections. Many of these people were the victims of physicians, nurses, and hospital workers who did not wash their hands. A 1999 study done at Duke University spotlighted the shocking reality that those of us who work in hospitals have observed for years: Many doctors and nurses do not wash their hands between patients. Yet hand washing is without a doubt one of the surest ways to prevent hospital-caused infection. One related study cited in the *Annals of Internal Medicine* (January 19, 1999) found that even among those doctors, nurses, and other hospital staff who do wash between patients, many don't do it long enough to be effective. Protocols require 30 seconds of hand washing; the study found many of these people washing for less than 10 seconds.

The problem for the patient is how to bring up the subject in a tactful but effective way. Rather than accuse anyone of being unhygienic, I'd say a good approach to take is to ask them to indulge you as a "Nervous Nellie." You could say something like, "I know you may think I'm a little paranoid, but I've been reading about the rise in hospital-caused infections, and I'd just feel a lot better if I could be assured that everyone's scrubbed before my procedure starts."

### Know what to expect when you awake from surgery.

In Chapter 3, I suggested that you ask your surgeon ahead of time to brief you on where you'll be and how you'll probably be feeling when you wake up from the anesthesia. If there's a big discrepancy between what you were told and what the reality turns out to be, find out the reason for it (that is, if you're up to asking for explanations); or let your patient advocate find out why your post-operative course is not going quite as anticipated. The box below provides a story in point.

---

**Peg woke up from knee surgery** to find her leg strapped into a machine that kept bending it slowly. "I was shocked!" she reported. "I asked the nurse what was going on. I thought I was going to rest after surgery, not exercise." It was 1989 and Peg's doctor was the best orthopedic surgeon she could find in the upstate New York city where she lived. She didn't realize—partly because she had never asked about her post-surgery therapy and partly because her doctor had not thought to brief her— that he would be using a brand-new technique that few other orthopedists had tried, and his familiarity with cutting-edge therapies had a lot to do with what made him "the best."

These days it's considered standard practice for certain types of post-orthopedic surgery patients to be put in the continuous passive motion machine (CPM) that Peg's orthopedist used then. But at the time, Peg thought he had gone too far. "I hate exercise!" she said. "I am not an athlete, and I told him to take me out of that thing and let me rest."

Her doctor tried lecturing her on the value of the CPM machine and how its use would accelerate her progress toward full recovery, but his talk came too late to do any good. "Get it out of here," she told him. The doctor pulled the plug on it.

---

If you awake from surgery with a very sore throat (and that's likely), ask if you can start doing saltwater gargles or have a throat lozenge. Most people complain that they have a sore throat after surgery under general anesthesia. To keep patients breathing during surgery, anesthesiologists use an *endotracheal tube* (a tube that goes all the way down the throat to the windpipe), which causes the soreness. Gargling with a gentle solution of warm saltwater or letting a numbing lozenge dissolve slowly in your throat will usually alleviate the problem until the pain goes away, typically in about a day. If you're not offered either of these remedies, just ask. (It's fine to spare your throat and make your request in writing!)

**If you wake up after surgery with a feeling of dry mouth but you are not yet able to drink, ask if you have a cup of ice chips to suck on.**
It may be a while after surgery before you are ready to eat or drink again, but in most cases, you'll be allowed to suck on some ice. Not only will ice chips relieve your dry mouth but if your throat is sore (and, as mentioned above, it probably will be) you'll find they also have a numbing, soothing effect on your throat.

**If you have a catheter, ask your surgeon and/or your nurse if it can be removed.**
A catheter is annoying at best and painful at worst, and leaving it in too long can lead to infection. Nevertheless, because they're so busy, hospital staff might leave it in longer than necessary. They just forget to check with your doctor to see when it's okay to remove your catheter—so ask about it. (And hope they don't utter in disbelief, "Oh my God, do you still have that thing in you?")

**Follow the same advice about IV lines, naso-gastric tubes, drains, and anything else you weren't born with.**
Ask if they can be removed yet. If the answer is no, ask when. If the answer is vague, keep asking until you get a definite answer. Don't let it slip anyone's mind that you'd like to be freed as soon as possible from these bodily invasions.

**If you're unsure about anything the nurse is doing, ask her to check to that your doctor has authorized it.**
Sometimes the nurses leave tubes and catheters in because they're following orders, so when you see your surgeon, be sure to check those

orders. Say, "Is having this thing in my body one more day really going to improve my care?" The answer may be "yes," but your question may also lead the doctor to take stock of your situation more frequently, and give you the answer you'd like, sooner rather than later.

**Tell your nurses and other health care providers how you prefer to be addressed.**
Once you're in your hospital room, you will find people coming to you at all hours with instructions, questions, and advice. They will begin every conversation with your first name, even though you've never met them before. If you're a laid-back sort of person who likes informality, that's fine—ignore this tip. But if you are a lady or a gentleman above a "certain age," you may well resent having some pimple-faced young medical student walk in and immediately call you "Pat." You should have no hesitation in saying, "Well, my oldest friends call me that, but I would really appreciate it if you would call me Mrs. Brown."

**Always go to the bathroom before your IV is started.**
Dragging an IV pole to the bathroom is awkward. If you see a doctor or nurse headed for you with the IV equipment, it's always worthwhile to make one last try to go to the bathroom.

**Know how to recognize the symptoms of *spinal headache* and ask for treatment of this painful side effect.**
A potential side effect of both spinal and epidural anesthesia is known as spinal headache, also called post-dural puncture headache. It's not a particularly common complication following an epidural injection, but it occurs just frequently enough that I believe patients should be warned to watch out for it. The headache results when the needle punctures the fluid-filled sac that surrounds the brain, the spinal cord, and its branches. The leak of spinal fluid leads to headaches when the patient is sitting or standing up. Sometimes the headache brings with it the companion problems of ringing in the ears, double vision, nausea or vomiting, or photophobia (sensitivity to light). A spinal headache will usually go away after a few days of bed rest, analgesics for pain, and plenty of coffee. The caffeine helps reduce the persistent ache.

Still, there's no need, in my view, to suffer through a day or two of any of these symptoms, treated only with these conservative measures, when there is a simple therapy available that will effectively remove their cause. All the anesthesiologist needs to do is "patch up the hole" with an *epidural blood patch.* During this procedure, the anesthesiologist essentially repeats the process of administering an epidural, but the patient's own blood is injected while the patient lies on his or her side in a comfortable position. The patient may also

---

***After a long, painful,*** and non-progressing labor, Lucy had a cesarean section that produced a beautiful baby girl. Her epidural allowed her to be awake during the procedure and see her healthy baby as soon as she was delivered. Lucy was glad that the baby was fine, but she soon discovered that she herself was not feeling well at all. In fact, she felt absolutely rotten. But never having had a baby before, she didn't know that the crushing headache she was experiencing was abnormal. Her obstetrician came to see her but didn't take note of Lucy's ashen face or look of pain and distress, nor did he think to ask her how she was feeling, generally. Fortunately, the pediatrician who came to check on both mother and baby was more observant.

"You look awfully washed out," he remarked. "Is anything wrong?"

Lucy didn't want to sound like a complainer, but she timidly mentioned the pounding in her head.

The pediatrician knew Lucy had recently had an epidural. "Must be a spinal headache," he concluded. "Let's get the anesthesiologist back. You'll get an epidural patch that will get rid of that headache completely."

Within the hour Lucy's headache was gone, and she could begin feeling comfortable with her new baby. She only wishes she had been warned about the possibility of spinal headache before the epidural started, so that she could have asked hours earlier for the relief she needed.

---

choose to sit upright for this procedure. The blood then clots and serves as a patch, preventing further leakage of spinal fluid through the puncture. The procedure isn't painful, but patients sometimes feel low-grade discomfort in the back or neck right after the injection. In the vast majority of patients, it cures the problem immediately, unlike the other conservative approaches.

In most cases your anesthesiologist won't know you're suffering from spinal headache and offer the patch unless you report the symptoms and request the treatment. As the story in the box on page 148 makes clear, you mustn't count on your surgeon to recognize your spinal headache for what it is or know how best to deal with it. By the way, you probably want to find out who pays the cost of the epidural blood patch. In many hospitals the patient isn't held financially liable for correcting this known complication of spinal or epidural anesthesia. But do check your bill to be sure you haven't been charged anyway.

### Watch for the side effects of narcotic pain medication.

If you're given any narcotic drugs for pain, let your doctor know if you have any of the following: constipation, trouble urinating, itching, nausea, and/or excessive drowsiness. These are all common side effects, and there are measures that can be taken to relieve them. A little anti-nausea medication, some clear juice, or maybe a glass of ginger ale—these are examples of simple comforts a nurse could provide for you. It could also be that you need your dosage adjusted downward, so make sure your doctor hears about any adverse side effects you are experiencing.

### Get more or different pain relief if you're still in pain after receiving a dose of your medication.

Don't accept the idea that there's nothing more that can be done. The range of pain medications available these days is broad and varied. If your medication isn't working for you, then your doctor should keep trying different dosages or drugs until something does. Some patients hate to complain; they just accept the fact that surgery is painful and grit their teeth and try to bear it as best they can. Some doctors, too, encourage this sort of attitude in their patients. Studies have found that under-medication of patients in pain is a widespread problem. One possible explanation is that doctors are afraid of becoming known to federal drug enforcement officials as someone who overprescribes or allows patients to abuse drugs. But patients have a right to effective pain relief. Newer, stronger drugs, such as Vioxx, Celebrex and OxyContin, can deliver relief for the majority of patients experiencing post-surgical pain. You may not be in condition to demand your right to effective pain treatment, but your patient advocate should certainly make this a top priority.

**If you experience mild nausea as a side effect of your pain medications, ask your doctor if you can use ginger products as a remedy.**
For severe or moderate nausea, let your doctor choose the most effective method of dealing with it, but if you're just feeling a certain queasiness after your pain pill takes hold, a bit of ginger may do the trick. Try sipping ginger ale or eating ginger-spiced foods or using ginger supplements (but only with your doctor's approval). This tip is applicable only for those allowed to eat and drink, of course.

**After surgery, when your doctor comes to see you, verify which medications you will be taking.**
They may not be the same as those discussed with you before surgery for any number of reasons, such as your response to the surgery or because of personal preferences you may have expressed to the anesthesiologist in your pre-surgery interview. Make sure your patient advocate is also aware of any changes in the medications you will be taking. Before you swallow a pill for the first time, take a moment to see what it looks like, so that you can recognize it the next time. When you know what drugs you expect to take, you'll be able to put the advice below into practice.

**When you are in the hospital, if you are given a pill that looks different from what you have been taking or expect to take, ask what the pill is before you pop it in your mouth.**
If you've followed the previous tip and learned what your medications

look like, you won't take just anything you're handed. Ask questions before you swallow, and if the answers don't reassure you, follow the tip below.

**When in doubt, say, "Wait. I'd like to speak with my doctor first to be sure this is something I'm supposed to have."**
This advice applies to more than pill-taking. It goes for tests, removal of sutures, new exercise instructions, and all other unexpected changes. If you will insist that hospital staff members verify what they are doing, you will go a long way toward protecting yourself from unnecessary or erroneous actions. (The story in the box on page 152 is a good example of a case calling for this precaution.) You will also help your doctor learn to be a good communicator (if she hasn't been all along) by making clear that you won't just go along with any hospital staff member's orders without first being informed about the reason for the change.

**Keep a copy of your list of medications and dosages handy as a reference for yourself, your patient advocate, and others involved in your care.**
In Chapter 3, I advised you to create a list of the drugs you take, the dosages, and the times. In Chapter 6, I suggested that you bring that list to the hospital with you. In one of the tips above, I said you should check with your doctor post-surgery so that your list can be updated to reflect any new drugs you are taking or to drop any drugs you have stopped taking now that your problem has been handled surgically. Don't assume, just because you are in a hospital, that your caregivers will always make sure you get only those medications your doctor ordered.

Errors in dosing and mix-ups of the medications to be given are far more common than they should be in most hospitals. Your best way to protect yourself is to have a written list of everything you're meant to receive and when. Keep your list where nurses and other hospital staff members can see it at all times—taped above your bed, for example. To protect the list from spills, you might even get it laminated.

## Post warning notices about drugs or other substances you need to avoid.

Let's say you can't use any drugs containing codeine. My suggestion is to write "No Codeine" on bright orange sticky notes. Put them on your bedside table, on your gown, on the bed frame. You might resent

***Addison's case of severe*** food poisoning had the infectious disease specialists at the hospital baffled. He'd had four inches of his large intestine removed during emergency surgery, necessitated by the perforation of his colon caused by food-borne toxins. The head of the infectious disease department came to visit. "You must come to the radiology department for a CT scan of your intestines," she told Addison.

He didn't think to question her about the necessity of the test. He was feeling weak and wrung out after the surgery, and he still had a high fever, despite having been on strong IV antibiotics around the clock. But he allowed himself to be put in a wheelchair and brought to the testing center, where he was subjected to the scan, which involved inflating his abdomen with fluid before taking multiple images of his insides.

The next day his surgeon came to visit. "Why did I have that test?" Addison asked. "It was incredibly painful. Couldn't it have waited till later?"

The surgeon was shocked. "I didn't order that!" he told Addison. "I would never have wanted you put through that in your condition! If I had known, I'd have put a stop to it." He went on to point out that the test wasn't to the patient's benefit at all. "The infectious disease department just wanted to satisfy their curiosity about the pathology." Then he added, "Next time, call me if anyone wants to do anything to you that I haven't told you would happen."

Too late for Addison—but I hope this tip will save some of my readers from similar trouble.

having to do this and think to yourself, "Why can't I assume that medical professionals will know to read my chart?" They probably will, but you want the extra protection for that slim chance that someone will slip up. I'm sure you've had the experience of being in a restaurant and asking to have an order done in a special way. You tell the waiter, "I'd like the salad dressing on the side, please," but when your salad is put in front of you and you take that first bite, you realize you've just had a mouthful of balsalmic vinaigrette. That kind of mistake is not such a big deal when it concerns a salad, of course. But it *is* a big deal in a hospital if the substance you've just ingested can cause a potentially deadly anaphylactic reaction—so don't worry about seeming overprotective. Your safety is a lot more important than a side order of dressing, and anything you can do to diminish the chance of an error is an effort well spent.

### Repeat your drug allergies to doctors, nurses, and pharmacists *every time* you receive a new medication.

This step is necessary, because if you have one drug allergy, you are very likely to be allergic to other related drugs. A common example of this problem concerns penicillin. An estimated 10 percent of people with a penicillin allergy also have an allergy to cephalosporins, antibiotics used to treat a wide variety of bacterial infections, such as respiratory tract infections, middle ear infections, skin infections, and urinary tract infections. Familiar cephalosporins, such as Keflex, could trigger a reaction, so if you have a penicillin allergy, at the very least, don't take your first dose of the medicine far away from an emergency room.

Don't assume, however, that you're allergic to a drug just because you experience some side effects after taking it. Your reaction could just be a sensitivity. For example, many people can't take aspirin because it irritates the stomach. That's a sensitivity, not a true allergic reaction. Of course, it's worth your while to make your sensitivities known, too. Two other indicators of a possible true aspirin allergy are polyps in the nose and allergic rhinitis. Those who must avoid aspirin frequently will be allergic to other non-steroidal anti-inflammatory drugs (NSAIDs), such as Naprosyn, as well. If you're not certain

---

**Checklist to Guard Against Medication Errors**

☐ Know the name of each medication you take—not just "a painkiller."

☐ Always ask when and how often each medication will be given to you.

☐ Know your proper dosage for each medication.

☐ Ask your patient advocate to help you keep track of the medications you receive. Ask him or her to write down all the information—the drug names, and how often, how much, and what times of day—and keep the list updated as your medications change.

---

whether your reaction is a drug allergy or sensitivity, then make your doctor aware of your experience with the suspect drug, or class of drugs, before you get your new prescription.

**Be on guard against common errors, such as doctors or nurses confusing you with another patient or thinking you've already had a test that never was performed.**

A doctor on hospital rounds typically rushes from one patient to another, glancing from chart to chart and monitor to monitor, while dispensing medications or issuing orders for them. It's not hard to see how mistakes can creep into the process, whether from the hurried doctor getting confused about the patient or the exhausted nurse getting confused about the doctor's orders. That's why you should *never* feel that speaking up with a question or objection about your medication is rude or out of place. You shouldn't have to suffer because of errors—and errors will be less likely to happen if you follow the rules in the checklist above.

**Make a special request for same-sex caregivers or other accommodations that are consistent with your needs and beliefs.**

For religious, cultural or psychological reasons, as a man or woman, you may want professionals of only the same gender to touch you.

**Sandy was a patient** with polycystic ovarian syndrome, a difficult to diagnose disease, which causes infertility along with many other uncomfortable symptoms. She'd already undergone several painful tests, including a hysterosalpingogram (injection of dye into her fallopian tubes, followed by X-ray) and an endometrial biopsy (scraping of tissue from the lining of her uterus for laboratory analysis). The only test she still needed was a diagnostic laparoscopy, which was to be carried out under general anesthesia.

Before she went to the hospital for the procedure, she had a consultation with the reproductive surgeon who was to perform it. He glanced quickly at her chart and then asked her the date of her last menstrual period. Sandy was astonished. Because of her disease, she had not had a period in years. She'd told the doctor about that on her first meeting with him and repeated it on every subsequent one, and yet he still didn't remember—nor, apparently, had he bothered to check her file. How could she have confidence that he was ordering the right tests for her in the right order if he forgot this very basic fact about her, she wondered. She went ahead and scheduled the laparoscopy, but had the results forwarded to another doctor, who was recommended to her by a former patient. She found herself feeling much better about her course of treatment, once she had a doctor who cared enough to recognize her and remember the outline of her case history.

Hospitals should respect your preference and meet your needs to the maximum extent possible. In fact, this is something that may heavily influence your choice of hospital. Of course, you must first make your special needs known to the administrators who assign nurses to your care. You should also make sure your caregivers are informed about any ceremonial jewelry, headdresses, or other accessories that you wear in accordance with the dictates of your religion or the traditions of your heritage. You may not be able to keep them on through

every phase of your hospitalization, but efforts can be made to minimize the time that you must have them off.

### Ask your doctor or a nurse exactly what surgical terms mean, so that you're not always wondering what people are talking about doing to you while you're under their care.

You hear your surgeon ask for something "stat" and, by his tone of
voice, you may correctly suspect it means "right away"—but you
may not be sure.

Doctors and nurses commonly throw around terms like this, not
intentionally trying to make it hard for you to follow their conversation, but just because they're in the habit of doing so. They
often forget or are unaware that you're listening and feeling confused or anxious about what they're saying. Even a term like "OR"
(operating room) that's familiar to most television viewers may
not be familiar to you, because you never got into *ER* or any other
hospital show.

There is a simple solution: Just ask these people what they mean.
Don't let them get away with any jargon or acronyms when it concerns your care. To get a bit of a head start in learning some hospital
language, you might want to check out the Glossary in the back of
this book. Also, take a look at Appendix C, which gives a sample
dialog between two doctors discussing a case, following by a "translation" into lay English.

### Do not accept condescending remarks.

When you ask questions, you deserve polite, informative answers,
not a snapped response like "It's on your chart." That's not good
enough, especially if you have reason to suspect that your chart
hasn't been kept up to date (a common problem in some hospitals). If
you want to be sure you're not ending up with a double dose of
your medication—and believe me, you *do* want to be sure of this—
then you must keep asking until you get a helpful answer. If necessary, have your patient advocate ask the question for you, or go to the
next highest level up the hospital chain of command and ask your
question (and be sure to read Chapter 10, "Working the System to

Get What You Need," which is all about who's who in the hospital)—and don't forget to report that you were brushed off the first time you asked.

## Don't tolerate a bad roommate.
I'm all for patients getting private rooms, but if the hospital is too crowded or if your budget really can't handle the extra expense, then you'll have to share a double. But that doesn't mean you have to be stuck with whatever awful roommate you get. No hospital patient should have to put up with someone who is loud and obnoxious, who continues to disrupt your sleep when asked politely to let you rest, or who makes hostile or offensive remarks. When you make your request to be moved under these circumstances, you should find the hospital quick to comply. If not, you will definitely need to appeal to a higher level in the hospital's chain of command.

## Don't remain in an awful room.
You need to take action if you find yourself in a room that makes recovery difficult. You shouldn't have to put up with broken furniture, flickering lighting, peeling paint, uneven heating, broken air conditioning, or nonworking plumbing. If the problem can't be fixed within a few hours, the solution is to move to a different room. It's the responsibility of the hospital to make sure you receive proper accommodations. The story in the box below tells what can happen when you speak up for your rights as a patient.

---

*My wife's mother* had a terrible case of asthma. Someone who was obviously disconnected from her case put her on a floor that was being repainted. After some time of struggling to breathe because of the fumes, she asked to be moved. She was told, "We don't have any other rooms available." For good reason, she was adamant that another room be found. The hospital had to move her to an "executive suite" so she could breathe. In other words, yes, there was a room.

---

### Ask for real coffee for breakfast if that's what you normally drink

If you're a regular, caffeinated coffee drinker and you don't have coffee in the morning at the hospital, you may get a withdrawal headache. Since you're going to be in discomfort already, why add to it? Conversely, the hospital may serve regular coffee by default, so if you are a decaf drinker, be sure to specify what you want.

### Make sure that your special food requirements and requests are being accommodated.

In Chapter 6, I suggested that you investigate your hospital food options. I hope you found out how to get the kind of food you require. The trouble is, you don't always get what you're promised—and sometimes you don't even get what the doctor ordered. If you're in condition yourself to complain, do so the moment you discover that your food delivery doesn't match what you expected to receive. If you're not up to it, this is definitely something for your patient advocate to tackle.

If needed, your doctor should be ready to support your dietary requirements, especially if you need diabetic-safe meals or heart-healthy choices. If you keep Kosher, your congregation's member services committee (or other group that visits the sick) might be willing to take over arrangements to assure you of getting the certified Kosher meals that meet your religious requirements.

### Understand the phenomenon of *sundowning*. Ask hospital staff to take steps to minimize its effects.

The hospital is a strange environment that can induce bizarre reactions in some patients. Sundowning (also called *ICU psychosis*) is a phenomenon that usually occurs in the early evening, when people normally settle down and relax. For many people, it's the most pleasant part of the day. In the hospital, though, this is the time of day when people start to lose track of who they are and where they are. They miss their family. They become more sensitive to the loss of dignity and control symbolized by an ugly, open gown, IV lines, and strangers poking and probing. They often become agitated, disoriented, confused, and even combative. Doctors can give them a sedative or antipsychotic medication to relieve the symptoms, but in extreme cases, a sundowning patient will need to be restrained.

The elderly, patients with Alzheimer's disease, those with extremely serious or terminal illnesses, or those who have experienced a severe trauma are more likely to be affected by this phenomenon than other patients.

When you first hear a sundowning patient moaning or screaming from a room down the hall, you may find it disconcerting or even frightening. Knowing about what you're hearing can help you stay calm. Of course, that's not going to help you sleep. Ask for sleeping aid, set up a white noise machine, or use earplugs at night—or all three.

If the problem occurs every night, ask your patient advocate to speak to the staff about taking actions to alleviate the sense of isolation and disorientation that may be affecting the patient or patients who become unhinged around sundown. Some of the things the staff can do include: keeping family members informed and involved in the care of the affected patient; making sure there are calendars and clocks available so that the patient can keep track of time; keeping the patient connected to the outside world with news and entertainment; and responding promptly when a patient first begins to get agitated with gentle reassurances and comforts to let him or her know that there are people all around who care and are there to help.

Though there is little that you can do to help other patients when they're sundowning, remember that the hospital staff are well trained to deal with the phenomenon and are doing the best they can.

### Continue to practice any mind-body techniques that have helped you in the past to overcome stress or pain.

If you have learned how to use any relaxation techniques or if you practice any exercises that you have found work to relieve stress or pain, check with your doctor about incorporating them into your recovery regimen. Most doctors will encourage their patients to do anything that's been helpful to them, as long as it does not conflict with standard medical treatment.

Hypnosis, biofeedback, music, meditation, visualization, psychological counseling, and a host of other nondrug therapies have worked for the patients I've seen. Some patients love to get lost in music and meditation. If you can fully engage your mind through tools such as these, you may be able to reduce your reliance on drugs that can bring unwanted side effects. It's well known that the human body has its own set of endorphins—the "runner's high" isn't fiction—that make you feel as if you're bulletproof.

I would caution, however, against taking up with any new, unfamiliar technique while you're in the hospital—stick with what you know has been good for you before.

### Periodically inspect your surgical wound for redness, swelling, discharge, or foul smell.

A bandage isn't supposed to hide a problem, it's supposed to protect the part from germs outside. Your doctor and the hospital will probably both give you copies of instructions about checking your wound after you go home. But you don't want to wait until you're home to learn to check your incision for problems. You also want to review the instructions before you leave the hospital, to be sure you understand what you're looking for and get answers to any questions you may have.

You may need to overcome your squeamishness if your wound is large or unsightly. In some cases, psychological counseling is helpful. In all likelihood, the hospital can connect you with a counselor if you raise the issue.

### Tell your orthopedic surgeon if your cast feels too tight; periodically examine your toes or fingers.

Just because your cast was put on by a professional doesn't mean it was put on correctly. A properly applied cast should never compromise blood flow. Look for the warning signs: discolored toes or fingers, tingling, swelling, or severe tightness under the ends of the cast. When you pinch your fingertip, does the blood return quickly to the nail bed? If you have a cast on your arm, does your wedding ring fit properly, or is your finger so swollen that it won't fit? (Actually, it's better to keep rings off your hands if you have a cast on your arm, but some people feel strongly about always wearing their wedding band, so swollen fingers can become a serious problem.)

Keeping your leg or arm elevated can help reduce swelling. Do that while you're waiting for your doctor to come and check your cast's fit.

To ensure your safety, some doctors will insist that you stay in the hospital the first night after you receive your cast, depending on the severity of your injury. They feel it is imperative that you are near immediate help if you experience swelling.

### Don't be shy about using your call button.

All hospital rooms are equipped with call buttons because that is the best way for patients to let nurses know when they need assistance. It's not an emergency system; you're probably hooked up to monitors that will sound an alarm if something's seriously wrong. The call button is there for you to use for your everyday needs: for example, your bedpan is full; you're thirsty but your water jug is empty; your pain shot is overdue; or you're chilly and could use an extra blanket. If you ring and no one comes after ten minutes or more, don't give up. Nurses do get busy, but don't let yourself be forgotten. Try again. If you find the response is consistently very delayed, that's something for your patient advocate to look into.

### If you have a legitimate complaint, don't be afraid to express it.

Some patients don't like being the center of fuss and bother. They say things like, "I don't want to be any trouble," and so they don't complain when the wrong meal is delivered to their room or when something spills and no one shows up for hours to clean up the mess. They think to themselves, "It's not an emergency; the staff have more important things on their minds." But in all likelihood, what's occupying the staff is tending to the complaints of those patients who are simply more vocal than others.

Your needs when you are sick *are* important, and you don't have to apologize for wanting them recognized. Of course, I'm assuming that you're not going to be pressing your call button ninety-nine times an hour! You know that getting butter on your toast when you asked for margarine isn't the same as getting the wrong antibiotic in your IV drip. The latter needs immediate action or else you could have a deadly allergic reaction; the former may be against your doctor's dietary orders, but you could fix that simply by eating your toast unbuttered. Still, you asked for margarine, and you should get it ... if not with this breakfast, then with the next. But you won't, unless you (or your patient advocate) will speak up for what you need.

### If you need more privacy or quiet, ask the head nurse to reduce the number of intrusions.

It's perfectly reasonable to request that only essential staff members be admitted to your room. The head nurse is more likely to be able to control the situation than your own doctor, so she's the one to field this request.

### When all else fails, use your doctor's home phone number.

In Chapter 6, I suggested that you ask your surgeon or attending doctor for a home number, as well as the office after-hours number. When you're in absolute agony, and you've pushed your call button over and over with no response, and your patient advocate has gone searching high and low for a doctor to take a look at you, and the interns and residents shake their heads and say they aren't authorized to do anything for you—that's the time to make the call. When all other paths have been tried and led you nowhere, you need to get hold of the one person who has the authority to change the orders in your case. You can't always count on the doctor's answering service to understand how great your need is and act as quickly as you want. The story in the box on page 163 is an excellent case in point.

*Glenda had just had* lung cancer surgery. She spent her first night in the hospital with her torso swathed all over in tight, heavy bandages. Although she was on pain medication, she could still feel every breath like a stab in her wounded lungs. What was worse, though, was the wetness and stickiness she felt all over her chest and back because her bandages were leaking. She rang for the nurse to change her bandage, but the nurse said it wasn't supposed to be done overnight. "Let me talk to a doctor," Glenda asked feebly.

The resident was summoned, but he just looked at her and shook his head. The dressing change needed to be authorized by her own doctor. Glenda's husband called the doctor's answering service and explained the situation. Apparently, the person who took the message was not impressed with the problem. Hours passed, and the doctor did not call back. All the while, Glenda was feeling more and more miserable. She started crying, then pleading and moaning, "Please, someone, just get me out of these wet bandages." Her husband was by now beside himself. He'd been married to her for forty years and had never seen her so distressed. Yet it seemed like such a simple thing she was asking for.

He rang again and again for the nurse. He tried reasoning with the resident. He tried yelling. That made things even worse. The resident got mad back, and threatened to call security to eject the husband from the hospital! None of this was doing Glenda any good.

Eventually the morning came, the night of hell was over, and she got her clean, dry bandages. Glenda needn't have suffered if only she had been able to get in touch with her doctor and get an order to have the bandage changed.

# CHAPTER 8

# When Your Child
# Has to Go to the Hospital

When your child is the one going to the hospital, you can and should still apply most of the advice in this book. You should meet with the surgeon and, if possible, the anesthesiologist, ahead of time and go over the child's health history and medication use thoroughly. You should know as much as you can about the procedure and the normal course of recovery, and you should be on the watch for complications and side effects of medications.

In some ways your job is easier, because you are the observer, not the patient—but in other ways it is much, much harder. Most parents would undergo almost any trauma themselves if by doing so they could spare their child from it. If your child is too young to understand or communicate effectively, it's doubly hard on you, because you see your child in pain after surgery and have to wonder, "Won't she blame her parents for bringing her here and putting her in this situation?" You know you want to be there every minute to cuddle her and let her know everything will be all right, yet the hospital's rules may keep you away at times. Still, children can and do emerge from hospital stays much better in both body and spirit than they went in. To boost the odds that your child will be one of them, I'm sure the tips and suggestions that follow will be of help.

### Ask the hospital to provide an orientation tour for you and your child.
Preparation can transform a potentially frightening experience for your child into an anticipated adventure. Pediatric hospitals, especially,

tend to give reassuring and informative tours. Usually the tour is conducted by a nurse—although it could be someone from the anesthesia department—who is friendly, outgoing, and good with kids. On the tour you and your child will be introduced to the staff members most likely to care for your child, and you'll become familiar with the places your child will be staying before, during, and after the procedure. I'd say an orientation tour is a great idea for almost all children, the only exception being those having a quick "in-out" procedure not involving general anesthesia or using any large and potentially scary machines.

**If the procedure will involve general anesthesia, make sure your child is fully prepared for the experience.**

If the hospital's orientation tour doesn't include a complete look at the way anesthesia is administered, then contact the anesthesia department separately and schedule an introductory visit. What's most helpful is giving your child a chance to see the mask that's used to administer anesthesia. In pediatric cases in most hospitals these days, your child will get a choice of flavors or scents to be sprayed on the mask to make it smell like a familiar treat. Choices may include bubble gum, orange, strawberry, grape, or other candy or fruit flavors. (Wonder why we don't have sprays in mint, charbroiled steak, Cuban cigar, and vodka martini for the adults?) Getting to choose a favorite flavor may not exactly turn an operation into fun, but it does give the child a bit of control over an important (to the child, anyway) part of the process.

Also, make sure that your child has ample time on the tour to ask any questions about how the anesthesia works. If you sense that your child hasn't grasped something or is confused, then restate what you've learned in terms you think your child will understand, checking with the tour leader to be sure you're putting things correctly.

**Review the informed consent form with your child's doctor to be sure it covers all actions you might conceivably want the doctor to take—or, if you prefer, is restricted to any specific actions you and the doctor have discussed.**

Sometimes a doctor will refrain from providing a certain service—a caudal block to treat post-operative pain, for example—because the consent form does not specifically cover it and its attendant risks.

If there is some specific treatment you want, and only that treatment, then by all means spell it out in the consent form for your child's procedure. However, if you have a good understanding of what your child's surgeon plans to do and want to leave him or her free to make judgment calls about your child's care as the surgical situation develops, then a broadly worded consent form will better serve your purposes.

**If your child is nervous or agitated or if the procedure will take many hours, ask the anesthesia department to provide your child with a liquid sedative before general anesthesia is administered.**

Most children need to be eased into the surgical experience. You can't expect them to react logically when they see the anesthesia mask coming down, even if you've explained to them over and over what it's for and why they need it. Many kids will panic, regardless of the amount of preparation they've had. You and your child's anesthesiologist need to have a plan in mind of what you will do if your child balks at being put under. You never want to let the doctor use brute force to put the anesthesia mask on your child's face. There is another way: Anesthesiologists can safely combine sedative medicines like Versed with a small amount of clear fruit juice or Tylenol elixir to give kids orally before using the mask. Versed also comes premixed in a cherry-flavored syrup for oral administration. By the time the doctor or nurse applies a mask for general anesthesia, these young patients are calm. Actually, they act like they've had a pitcher of margaritas. Parents see the result and sometimes joke that they'd like to take a vial of the stuff home "for those bedtimes when you just can't get them to settle down."

In some cases the child's fear is so strong that he or she will refuse to drink the elixir. If that happens, one option is for the doctor to give your child a very quick and relatively painless shot of sedative in his rear end. It is better for your child to feel a little sting and relax quickly, than to be fully awake and traumatized by the anesthesia mask coming down.

### Make sure you are allowed to stay with your child as anesthesia is being administered.

It used to be rare for hospitals, even pediatric facilities, to allow parents into the OR. Now it's widely accepted that parents belong with their children during the start of surgery, and it's understood that when children have a parent's reassuring presence, they are far less anxious and more likely to go into surgery with a positive outlook. Studies comparing results in children who were separated from their parents with children who were allowed to have parents with them have shown little doubt that outcomes are better when parent and child go in together.

### Find out if you can be in the recovery room as your child is waking up.

Here you will find hospital policies vary greatly. Most will not allow parents to come into the recovery room. The reason for the policy is to allow the doctors and nurses the time and space they need to monitor the child's post-surgical progress without anxious parents hovering around. The parents might be invited into the recovery room just as the child is being wheeled out, but some hospitals stick with the old rule that parents can see their child only after the child is moved to a hospital room. Although you'll probably want to be with your child the moment he or she is awake, keep in mind that after general anesthesia patients (of any age) tend to be in a fog, and even if they're aware of your presence at the time, they're very likely to lose the memory of it by the time they're fully awake, several hours later.

### If you learn that you can't be in the recovery room as your child awakes, make sure your child is aware of that.

Whatever the hospital's policy about parents in the recovery room, make sure your child knows what to expect. If the procedure is done under a local anesthetic and your child is conscious the whole time, but you're not permitted to be there, you don't want your child crying the whole time, "Where's Mommy? Where did Daddy go?" Young children can often accept calmly what their parents tell them is fact, but it's sometimes much harder for them to deal with any sort of abrupt change, something not going according to what they've been led to expect. If you don't show up at a time when your small child thinks you're supposed to be there, he or she might assume you've disappeared for good. So if you're not going to be with your child at any point when he or she will be awake, say so, but then quickly let your child know when you *will* be there. Ask a nurse who's established a good relationship with your child to provide reassurance that she'll be taking good care of him or her all the while, and that you will be back as soon as you possibly can.

## Use videotapes and books to familiarize and reassure your child about his or her hospital stay.

One videotape that I recommend is *A Hospital Trip with Dr. Bip,* produced by KiDz-Med. It's available in English and Spanish and can be ordered over the Internet (*www.kidzmed.com*) or by contacting KiDz-Med at 305-361-6378.

There are lots of books for children about the hospital experience. Most are aimed at young children who can't yet read on their own. You can get books written about familiar characters, like Paddington Bear *(Paddington Bear Goes to the Hospital),* Franklin the Turtle *(Franklin Goes to the Hospital),* or Curious George *(... Goes to the Hospital).* There's also a book by Fred Rogers—that is, "Mr. Rogers" of the preschool-age TV show—called *Going to the Hospital.*

But before you read any book to your child or show a videotape, I'd suggest you review it first. That way you can be prepared to deal with any questions you think the book might provoke, or perhaps fast forward through any part of the tape that is irrelevant to your child's case, or that your child might find confusing.

## Make room for blankies and teddies.

You should definitely pack these items. If at all possible, your small child should be allowed to hold the comforting object while being sedated. As soon as you are allowed to reunite with your child, bring the blankie or teddy bear back to your child. You might also look into having a child's favorite blanket washed with a disinfectant detergent (if it can be done without shrinking or discoloring the material) so that there's no worry about the blanket bringing in germs.

### Be honest about pain while still staying upbeat and focused on the long-term benefits of the procedure.

There are books and articles that advise parents on how to talk to children about impending surgery. I'll recommend a book below, but first let me pass along a piece of advice that I think most child psychologists would endorse: Don't tell your child "it won't hurt a bit" when that's not true. You may calm your child's fears ahead of time, but you'll soon be unmasked as a liar. You don't want to buy short-term reassurance at the cost of long-term trust. On the other hand, you don't want to be too blunt and scare your child unnecessarily. You want your child to know that you'll do everything within your power to see to it that things are made as painless as they can be. You'll probably rely on euphemisms to a certain extent, words that soften the reality but do not mislead. For example, I'd avoid talking about stitches, which children naturally associate with sewing and with needles. The image of a needle and thread going back and forth through skin will be a painful one in the minds of most children, no matter what you say about the numbing medicines that will be used. And you definitely don't want to talk about staples, because kids can all too easily imagine what it would feel like to use a stapler on themselves. Instead, just talk about "closing." Whatever the doctor uses to close the wound is going to be covered with a bandage, anyway. Your child isn't going to get a good look at it for quite a while afterward, when the worst is long past.

Here is a book that may be useful when it comes to the task of discussing pain and other difficult issues: *Your Child in the Hospital: A Practical Guide for Parents* by Nancy Keene, Rachel Prentice, and Linda Lamb (O'Reilly & Associates).

### Ask the hospital to use *EMLA* on your child's skin to allow for painless IV starts.

EMLA, which stands for eutectic mixture of local anesthetics (the local anesthetics are lidocaine with prilocaine), is a white cream used to prevent pain. Applied about 45 minutes in advance of a procedure, it takes the sting and pain out an IV start, skin laser surgery, injections, and so on. It's an especially useful tool in raising the comfort level for a child in a hospital, but adults like it, too. In Chapter 4, "All about Anesthesia," I recommended that adults ask for an injection of lidocaine before an IV start, but I prefer EMLA for children, even though it doesn't take effect as quickly, because it's administered in the form of a cream, not a shot.

Most hospitals stock EMLA, but if you find out it's not available at your child's hospital, you should certainly ask your pediatrician to write a prescription for it. You can bring it to the hospital or, following your doctor's instructions, apply it to your child's skin at home ahead of time.

### Work with your child's doctor to find the best form of medication for your child.

Some children love the flavored syrups used as a base for many pediatric antibiotics. Others gag and choke with each dose. Some children learn to swallow pills by age four or five; others don't have the skill to do so until much later in childhood. Sometimes medicines can be combined with fruit juices or applesauce; if that turns out to be feasible with the ones your child needs, your doctor will let you know. As long as you achieve the goal of getting your child to take the full dose, the delivery method shouldn't matter. The point is to know your own child and provide your child's doctor with your best insights into your child's likely reactions to different possible methods of drug administration. What you're hoping to avoid is a situation in which nurses are holding your child down and forcing medicine down her throat every four hours. A little advance thought and perhaps experimentation with different medication delivery methods could make all the difference for your child.

### Tell the doctor "no surprises" as much as possible.

In order for you to prepare your child for the hospital experience, first your child's doctor has to properly prepare *you*. Although there may be a few times when a doctor or nurse must act quickly and without warning in your child's case, such instances tend to be limited to emergencies. In a scheduled pediatric procedure, it's more likely that the surgical team will have years of experience with children just like yours, and will be more than able to anticipate all the major complications that could arise. They should be able to give you a very complete picture of what is likely and unlikely to happen during the procedure.

You may not want to repeat every detail to your child, but keep your descriptions general, and pegged to your child's level of comprehension. Just cover all the major possibilities, so that your child isn't caught completely off guard—which is what happened to me when I had to go to the hospital at age twelve (see the story in the box below).

---

***When I was twelve,*** I broke my wrist. At the hospital, a doctor who was a friend of my dad's was going to take care of me. He and my dad spent a couple minutes talking in the corner, and when I saw my dad, I thought, "Why does he look so sad? It's just a broken wrist. He'll put a cast on it and all my friends will sign it. This is okay."

I didn't know that the doctor had to set the bone before the cast was put on my wrist. They were talking about whether to put me to sleep to set the bone or pull a "sneak attack" on me and set the bone without anesthesia.

My father looked dour, while the other doctor came over to me in a buddy-buddy way and said, "Dave, my boy, let me see this arm for a minute." Then he twisted my arm! My father turned the other way because he understood how much it hurt. I called this doctor every name in the book! I yelled, "Are you crazy?" And then I turned to my father and said, "Dad, why didn't you stop him?" My dad said he was sorry, but that it was the easiest, safest way to set the bone.

This experience was traumatic, and as a result I believe that every child in the hospital should be spared the "sneak attack."

---

**Maintain as much of your child's normal routine as possible.**
Try to keep babies or toddlers on their nap schedules if you can. Bring familiar foods, if allowed. Once your baby is eating solid food, it's hard to see why she shouldn't have the particular brand of strained peaches she likes brought from home, rather than jars off the hospital caterer's supply shelves. Anything you can do to reduce the strangeness of the situation and give the child some sense of familiarity and control over her surroundings will be a good thing.

**Expect some backward steps.**
Your three-year-old may have been mostly toilet trained, but it's normal for a hospitalized child to regress and go back to wetting or soiling the bed. Hospitals are set up to handle these kinds of accidents easily—there's no need to make a fuss. It's certainly no time to yell at your child or express any disappointment. Former thumb suckers usually start sucking again—and that's fine: any little comfort will help. In fact, I'd be more inclined to worry if the child did *not* act up in some way. It might indicate that the child was actually numb with fear, that is, simply too terrified to react in any way at all.

**Bring games to play with your child, and books to read, and think of stories to tell.**
Games, books, and stories are all great distractions, taking your child's mind off the realities of hospitalization and transporting both of you to an imaginary world where things are more fun. Just be sure you're not choosing intense games that require a high level of concentration or that get so heated that your child's stress level goes up. And avoid scary or gory books or stories. For older children, you might want to bring books on tape, which the child can control with a personal stereo system with headphones.

**Involve other relatives, caregivers, and friends in your child's hospital experience, if you can.**
One of the most frightening aspects of being in the hospital for a child is being cut off from familiar faces. Yes, you and your spouse will be there as much as you can, but your child still will miss seeing

school friends and aunts and uncles and grandparents and sitters. It's important to reassure your child that all these people care deeply and will be there for your child the minute he or she is home. Of course, if they can visit, that's wonderful (but see the caution below about child visitors). Cards, however, almost always help to brighten a child's day—as do balloons bouquets and baskets of cookies. Just be sure to check with your doctor to find out if your child can eat any treats that are sent in; you definitely don't want to show your child a giant cookie with "Get Well Soon" spelled out in pink frosting and then have to tell your child she can't touch it!

### Be cautious about letting other children visit your child— including the child's siblings.

First, you may find that the hospital's visiting rules restrict children to immediate family. But you should think through the pros and cons of bringing your child's siblings, especially if they're very young. After surgery, children may have tubes sticking out of their noses or needles taped to their arms. They almost certainly will look pale and small and dwarfed by all the monitoring machines and other bedside paraphernalia. You may fully describe the scene in advance and re-mind the young visitor not to say anything rude, but some kids just can't stop themselves from blurting out, "EEEWWWW, you look so *gross!*" Even children as old as eleven or twelve may find themselves unable to hold their first reactions in check. Actually, lots of adults blurt out the wrong things on hospital visits, too, and so let me amend this advice to say, invite only those visitors to the hospital that you're sure will be good at brightening your child's day.

### Become your child's patient advocate.

Read over the advice in Chapter 5 with a special eye for all the issues and problems the patient advocate should be ready to take on. Obvi-ously, your child won't be able to watch out for his or her own good. As a parent, that's your job. The hospital staff may be top-notch and very caring, but they are busy, and occasionally even the best can slip up. It's one thing if you, as an adult, miss a dose of your medication or your naso-gastric tube is left in too long—you can deal with that—

but it's quite a different thing when it concerns your child. You won't waste a minute in seeing that the situation is corrected and things are put right. Where your child is concerned, there's almost no such thing as an overprotective parent.

# CHAPTER 9

# When You Have No Time to Plan: Advice for Emergency Room Patients

This chapter starts out with some things you should know about emergencies in general—the kind of knowledge it's good to have in your head long before you have occasion to need it. You'll have extra peace of mind if you can be assured that the responsible adults around you (both at home and at work) are similarly knowledgeable, because when you're the one in need of an ambulance, you may not be in shape to tell others what you want them to do for you.

The chapter goes on to offer tips and suggestions for things to do once you arrive and while you're waiting, plus tips on ways to avoid being made to wait too long, as well as some advice about dealing with a few practical details, such as keeping track of your things after you've been admitted and giving notice to others that you've had an emergency.

**Know what kinds of problems call for an emergency room visit, so that you only go when you really need to.**
You should go to the emergency room if you are experiencing any of the following:

- Difficulty breathing, severe shortness of breath.
- Signs of a heart attack, including: pain across the chest or under the breastbone; pain radiating outward or up from the chest (down an arm or up the neck, especially); a sensation of squeezing or pressure in the chest, especially if accompanied by lightheadedness or dizziness.

- Signs of a stroke, including: suddenly going numb or feeling weak in the face, arm, leg, or on one side of the body; sudden loss of vision (may be in just one eye); loss of speech; trouble talking or understanding; a sudden, severe headache (in someone who doesn't usually have headaches or migraines); confusion or unsteadiness, especially when accompanied by any of the other symptoms listed above).
- Suspected poisoning—but always call your local poison control center first, because certain poisons should be vomited up as soon as possible, while others should be immediately diluted with water. Knowing what to do at home could save your life. If you don't already have the number of a local poison control center on a readily available emergency information sheet, you can call the 24-hour national poison control hotline at 1-800-222-1222.
- A severe or worsening allergic reaction (to a medication, an insect sting or bite, a food, or a contact substance), characterized by spreading hives and/or swelling of the tongue or airway.
- Any major injury, but especially one to the head or neck, one that leaves you with blurry or double vision, or one that has knocked you unconscious (even if only for a short time).
- Severe abdominal pain, especially when accompanied by a fever of 102 degrees or higher in an adult, 105 degrees or higher in a child.
- Unexplained stupor, drowsiness, or disorientation.
- Coughing up or vomiting blood.
- Bleeding that does not stop after 10 minutes of direct pressure.
- Any cut deep enough to warrant stitches.
- Broken bone (or suspected broken bone).

The next tip discusses whether or not to take time to call your doctor before you go.

**Call your doctor first—unless there's no time to spare.**
Whenever possible, you should notify your doctor before going to the emergency room. When every second counts—as it does when you're having a heart attack or not breathing well enough to talk—you'll skip this step, of course. It's still a good idea to have someone else call your doctor for you, if you can. That way, while the ambulance is taking you to the hospital, your doctor can be on standby to consult with the emergency room staff about your history and any treatment he or she would like you for to receive (or avoid, in some cases).

If you're able to make the call yourself, make sure the person answering the doctor's telephone hears the word "emergency." Otherwise, you might not get a call back until the doctor's regular hour for returning calls, which could well be at the end of the day. If it's already after business hours, then call your doctor's emergency number or answering service number. Say it's an emergency and briefly describe your symptoms. (See the tip later in this chapter about using the right terms to describe your emergency). Ask for an immediate call back, but don't wait around for it if your condition is unstable and possibly life-threatening; give a cell phone number if you have one. If you haven't heard back from the doctor before you're out the door, you might want to call the doctor's answering service back, just to say which emergency room you're going to. That way, your doctor can call to consult with the emergency room doctors about your care.

When a doctor phones in advance of a patient's arrival, the patient will usually be able to skip some of the hospital paperwork, and the ER staff will be better prepared to treat the patient. Your doctor may even suggest meeting you at the emergency room so that he or she can oversee your care personally. This is commonly the case when a patient calls his cardiologist to say he's having symptoms of a heart attack or when a pregnant woman lets her obstetrician know she's bleeding, experiencing premature contractions, or having some other signs of a serious problem with her pregnancy.

**Know when to call an ambulance and when to be driven.**
If you are in danger of losing consciousness, are bleeding profusely, or are in severe pain, then it's not safe for you to drive. Either call

an ambulance or accept a ride from someone on the spot, but do *not* call a taxi and wait. The box below gives some guidelines for emergency transport.

---

**Call an ambulance if**

- You should be moved only by medically trained personnel because of a possible back or neck injury.
- You need CPR (cardiopulmonary resuscitation) or oxygen.
- You are having convulsions or a seizure.
- You need someone to stop the bleeding.

**You can be driven if**

- You are in pain but are clear-headed (no double vision, no confusion, you know where you are and what happened to you).
- The pain comes and goes.
- You have experienced the symptoms before and know what treatment you need and know how soon you need it.
- You've spoken to your doctor and have been told you don't need to call an ambulance.

*Note:* If you are well enough to drive yourself, then it's probably not an emergency, and you should consider waiting until regular office hours to see your doctor.

---

**Bring your insurance information with you.**
You don't want to be scrambling to find your insurance information as you're being loaded into the ambulance, so always keep it in the same, easy-to-remember spot. Your wallet is the usual place.

Make sure your next-of-kin, partner, or roommate has a copy of the information, too. If you're in a boating accident and your purse has gone overboard, you don't want your hospital admission held up while your mother is tracked down and she tries to remember whether or not you switched health plans since you left your last job.

If you imagine that the hospital emergency room will just go ahead and do what's necessary to treat you and worry about the insurance details later, think again. Although the ER staff is supposed to act this way, there's no shortage of cases on record in which they've behaved in just the opposite manner. People do still get turned away from emergency rooms because they have no proof of insurance. This practice is called "dumping," and although it's been illegal since 1985 when Congress passed the Emergency Medical Treatment and Labor Act, hospitals can still get away with it by claiming that your condition did not meet the criteria for a medical emergency.

If you think your insurance company will waive its own hospital authorization requirements in an emergency—well, that could happen, but then again, it might not. Most insurance companies will still expect your emergency contact to jump through all the insurance pre-certification hoops for you. In any case, you don't want to have to worry about that possibility as you're being wheeled into the ER on a gurney—especially when the solution is as simple as making a photocopy of your insurance card and giving it to the person you've named as your emergency contact.

### Carry a card that details all medications you currently take and treatments you're undergoing.

You don't have time to prepare this in an emergency. This is something I recommend that everyone carry with them in their wallet at all times. Keep it updated as needed. Here's how to make the card:

Put all your pill bottles in front of you, including those of vitamins, herbs, and other supplements you take regularly. On a blank piece of paper set up three columns: one for "Name" (either brand name or generic name), one for "Dosage" (how many milligrams or micrograms in each pill), and one for "Schedule" (how many times a day you take the pill). If you're using a computer, choose a clear, clean font like Arial and a very small type size (8- or 9-point); the goal is to fit all the information within a $3^1/2$ by 2-inch space, the size of a credit card. If it doesn't all fit on one card, create a second, third, or fourth. Buy laminating sheets from an office supply store, and cut the card out and laminate it. If you've made two cards, laminate them front to back to create one double-sided card. If you've made four, then tape the two double-sided laminated cards together at the top, so that you have one fold-over card with all your drug information on it. Keep this card in your wallet right next to your health insurance card and your emergency contact information card. For an example of what the card should look like, see the box below.

### Sample Medication Card

| Name | Dosage | Schedule |
|------|--------|----------|
| Zantac | 75 mg | 2 x |
| Lipitor | 20 mg | 1 x |
| Ambien | 10 mg | 1 at bedtime |
| Multivitamin with iron | 30 mg of iron | 1 in a.m. |
| Calcium | 500 mg | 3 x |
| | | |

**Keep your medical history handy, with all your doctors' names and telephone numbers.**

This won't fit on something the size of a credit card, of course, so use full-size sheets of paper. List each doctor's name, specialty, office telephone number (main and alternate) and after-hours or emergency numbers. Under each doctor's heading you should list each medical condition or illness for which you are currently receiving treatment or for which you have undergone treatment within the past ten years. To be sure you are not leaving out anything affecting a major organ or organ system, it may help you to consider this list:

- Lungs: persistent breathing problems, serious respiratory illness, asthma, infection
- Heart and circulatory system: heart attack, congenital defects, arrhythmia, high cholesterol, hardening of the arteries

- Kidneys: infections, failure
- Digestive: colon problems, GERD (gastroesophageal reflux disease), ulcers
- Neurological: concussion, nerve damage
- Immune system: many skin disorders, AIDS, Raynaud's disease, rheumatoid arthritis
- Serious allergies, such as to penicillin or other medications
- Any other diseases that affect your long-term health.

Include in your listing of illnesses and conditions any operations or hospitalizations that were part of your treatment, followed by the date, or your best recollection of the date. You don't have to bother with minor matters, such as wart removal or correction of an ingrown toenail. I recommend you go back at least ten years when listing hospitalizations.

A good place to keep this document is tacked up on a corkboard or stashed in a mail holder or file by the telephone that you'd most likely use to call an ambulance or your doctor. That way, if you should find yourself dialing 911 or your doctor to report an emergency, you can grab your information and have it ready to take with you. If someone else is doing the calling, you can say, "Look in the mail holder right next to the phone. There's a red envelope in the last slot that has my medical information in it. I need to bring that with me." Using a brightly colored envelope is a good way to make the document easy to identify; you should also write your own name and telephone number in big letters and numerals across the top.

**Wear a medical alert bracelet if you have any medical problems that might leave you suddenly unable to communicate.**
Conditions that merit a medical alert bracelet are: diabetes; epilepsy; asthma; heart condition, allergies to penicillin or other medications; severe allergies to foods or other substances (for example, a peanut allergy; a strawberry allergy, an allergy to latex products).

Another condition that I believe merits a medical alert bracelet is difficulty with intubation. If you've ever been intubated before and were told by the staff afterward that there was a problem getting the tube down your throat, you would be well advised to make that fact known in an emergency. Then, if you ever need to be rushed into surgery, your operating room staff will know that they must treat you differently. You will give them the information they need to keep you breathing.

The medical information bracelet most commonly seen is the one produced by the Medic Alert Foundation (2323 Colorado Avenue, Turlock, CA 95382; toll-free telephone number: 888-633-4298; website: *www.medicalert.org*). Once you have joined the organization and ordered the bracelet with the appropriate medical warning, a computer file containing your doctor's telephone numbers and important details about your medical history is created for you at the Medic Alert monitoring center. When *emergency medical technicians (EMTs)* see a Medic Alert bracelet, not only do they know what condition you

---

*Catherine got a call* one afternoon at her home in Washington, D.C., from the manager of a small airport in central Florida. He said, "Your husband is down here acting crazy. If you don't come and get him soon, I'm afraid we may have to have him locked up." Catherine said the entire event almost spiraled out of control, because it took the manager so long to find her: "My husband had a history of mental illness. He had been on a trip, but had forgotten to take his medication. At the first sign of a problem, if someone had been able to find out where he was from and whom to contact in an emergency, I would have been able to say, 'Just make him take his pills.' But all they found that had any identifying information was the pills themselves with the number of the VA hospital in Washington, D.C. They had to call the hospital, and somebody who answered had to locate his doctor, and his doctor had to go through his records to find my number. It took hours."

Now Catherine makes sure that wherever her husband goes, he keeps a card in his wallet naming her as his emergency contact.

---

have, but they can also call the monitoring center and find out how to reach your doctor and learn other facts about you that will help you to receive the right treatment without delay.

### One more essential piece of information you need in your wallet is your emergency contact information.

Type on a piece of paper the name of the person you want notified in case you are unable to speak for yourself in an emergency. Tell the person's relationship to you (spouse, parent, sibling, domestic partner). List home address and telephone number and all other likely contact numbers, including office, cell phone, and/or pager. Cut the paper so that it is credit-card sized and laminate both the front and back. You might want to use a small piece of tape to attach the card on one side to your health insurance card, so that if anyone goes looking for your health insurance information, they'll discover your emergency contact card at the same time. To see a sample emergency contact card, see page 257 in Appendix A.

The story in the box on page 184 tells what can happen (and all too often does happen) when this information is not available.

### Patients under treatment by multiple doctors should ask that all of them be notified of your emergency admission and kept up on details of your treatment.

Until electronic medical record keeping improves, coordinating care among various doctors will continue to be very difficult, so be prepared to help them out. Certain diseases, AIDS and many forms of cancer among them, require the cooperation of multiple specialists to deliver the best care to the patient. Older patients who tend to have a number of concurrent medical conditions also fit this category.

When you're on the way to the hospital, you normally won't have time to make multiple phone calls. If you've brought the names and numbers of all of your doctors with you, the ER nurse may contact them for you. A different approach would be to ask your primary care physician to be your medical care coordinator. When you're taken to the hospital, you make sure your primary care physician has been called; he or she then knows who your other doctors are and will notify them about your admission and consult with them on your treatment as needed.

### Know what to expect when you arrive: Understand the *triage* system used in emergency rooms.

"Triage" comes from the French word for "sorting," which is exactly what ER nurses and doctors do to each arrival at their doors. They quickly assess who needs immediate attention, who can wait a short while, and who can safely be seen once all the other urgent and middle priority cases have been taken care of. No emergency room is "first come, first served." The ideal is "greatest need, first served."

The trouble is that nurses and doctors don't always accurately assess whose need is greatest. Sometimes a stoic, quiet patient with internal bleeding will not receive attention ahead of a highly agitated patient with what turns out to be a bad case of indigestion. Studies have shown that women with heart attack symptoms are more frequently sent home from emergency rooms than men who report the same symptoms. Much depends on three factors: the skill of the person making the initial assessment, the way the patient's measurable symptoms (blood pressure, temperature, appearance, and other indicators) match up with the correct emergency diagnosis, and the ability of the patient to communicate what's wrong clearly and effectively.

The next three tips are intended to help with each of these three factors in turn.

### Know which emergency room in your area is the best at what you need.

No one can "shop around" during an emergency, so this is something to take care of when you have no special reason to think you'll be needing to visit an ER soon. A good place to start is with your primary care physician. Ask her opinion of the quality of care at the various emergency rooms in local hospitals, starting with the one nearest you. (Closeness is definitely an important factor, though by no means the only one.) If you see a specialist for a problem that has the potential to become an emergency, ask that specialist which emergency room she likes to send her patients to.

***Maryann once had*** an allergic reaction to the drug Flagyl, which she had been taking to combat a parasitic infection picked up while swimming in some unnamed body of water. Before taking the drug she had read the precautionary notes about stomach upset, diarrhea, loss of appetite, nausea, dizziness, and headache. One by one, she got the nasty reactions to some degree and coped with them. However, when her symptoms expanded to include rash, hives, painful urination, mouth sores, and tingling in her hands and feet, she knew she had to do as the package warning sheet directed and seek immediate help. By the time she got to the emergency room, she had a full body rash. The triage staff knew at once to check her for breathing problems—the next stage in a progressively bad reaction to the drug. Being taken in ahead of others in the ER waiting room was a sure sign that her condition was indeed urgent. If Maryann had ever doubted she needed hospitalization, the doubt was erased by being bumped to first place in the triage system.

Another factor is ease of transportation. If the emergency room is just a couple of miles away but getting there means crawling through bumper-to-bumper traffic, you might be better off going to one that's slightly farther out but on a faster route. Even ambulance drivers can't make clogged streets flow freely.

Also consider the type of emergency you have. When a child is the patient, you want an emergency room in a hospital that has a pediatric department—even better would be the emergency room of a pediatric hospital. If there is time, consult the child's pediatrician and take the child where you are directed. The same advice applies when choosing an emergency room in case of a possible heart attack, or if you think you've broken a bone. The staff at the specialized hospital will usually have the advantage when it comes to speedy diagnosis and appropriate treatment.

Time and place can also affect your choice of where to go. If your emergency occurs on a Saturday night, I'd say, as a general rule, you should avoid a downtown emergency room. Saturday nights are club-hopping and partying nights, and that's when urban emergency rooms tend to get crowded. People come in having overdosed on drugs, or they have alcohol toxicity from binge drinking, or they've been in fights or accidents, or they've been shot. Unless your complaint has dramatically apparent and life-threatening symptoms, you're probably going to be in for a long wait in a downtown emergency room. Marty's story in the box on page 189 is in many ways typical.

My advice is to do a bit of research about emergency rooms while you're still healthy. Try checking the annual index of your local consumer ratings magazine to find out if any articles have been published comparing the emergency rooms in your area. You could also go to the library or newspaper archives to see if your local paper has ever done a piece investigating the emergency care available in the region. There's also informal research you can do: Simply ask your friends and neighbors about their experiences at the different emergency rooms. People usually like to give their opinions and, if they've had a bad experience somewhere, warn you away from the place that treated them badly.

**Help the ER staff assess your condition accurately by understanding their questions and by providing precise answers.**
There's a mnemonic for the series of questions that EMTs ask victims when assessing their pain, which goes by the alphabetical abbreviation PQRST. If your emergency involves pain, you can expect to be asked the PQRST questions below.

- ✓ *Provokes*—What causes the pain? What makes it better? What makes it worse?
- ✓ *Quality*—What does it feel like? Is it sharp? Dull? Stabbing? Burning? Twisting? Crushing?
- ✓ *Radiates*—Where does it radiate? Does it start in one place and go someplace else? Down your back? Up your neck? Down your arm? Or leg? Is it all in one spot? Did it start in one place but now it's mainly in another location?
- ✓ *Severity*—On a scale of 1 to 10, with 10 being the worst, how do you rate it? Is it always that bad, or does it get better or

**Marty, who is in** his mid-twenties, has been to the emergency room twice in his life. The first time, he had broken his ankle when he slipped on some stairs going down to the basement of his apartment building in an urban neighborhood of Washington, DC. His friends drove him to the nearest emergency room, less than a mile away. It was on a Saturday night, and a broken ankle, Marty quickly realized, just wasn't enough of a problem to get him seen anytime soon—not when the waiting room was as crowded as it was with car accident victims, screaming psychotics having hallucinations, and shooting and stabbing victims arriving by ambulance one after another. Marty waited for hours, but not all that time was wasted. He learned something valuable in the process. Next time, he'd go elsewhere.

A few years passed. It was another Saturday night and Marty had made dinner for a few friends. He was slicing bread with a large, very sharp knife when his hold on the knife slipped and he sliced his hand deeply. Fortunately, one of his guests was a doctor (a psychiatrist, as it happened) who knew what to do to stop the bleeding. "That cut needs stitches," his guest told him, adding that cuts in the hand, if not stitched up within an hour or two, will not heal properly. Movement can be permanently impaired.

Marty already knew that the closest emergency room was not the place to go for speedy treatment of minor injuries. He knew of another hospital with an emergency room in the close-in suburbs. It was far less likely, Marty figured, to be filled with victims of the Saturday night downtown party scene. He had his friend drive him four miles to that ER. As predicted, it was quiet: The only other patient behind the curtained area was an elderly woman being treated for a possible heart attack. Not only was Marty stitched up quickly, but the initial ER doctor called in a plastic surgeon to do the work, to be sure that Marty had the least visible scar.

worse? How bad is it when it's at its worst? At its most tolerable? How long do the bad episodes last? When it's at its worst, are you forced into a particular position (lying down or sitting up)?

✓ *Timing*—When did it start? Was it sudden or gradual? What were you doing at the time? Has it ever happened before? How often do you experience it?

Your answers to these questions will lead the person assessing you to ask certain follow-up questions to elicit even more detail from you about your condition. It's important not to get impatient or insist that your questioner get right to the particular problem you believe should be addressed. There is a reason why questions are asked in a particular sequence. Issues that may seem off-target to you still need to be explored, to rule possible diagnoses and complications in or out. By listening carefully to the questions and providing all the details you're asked for, you will help the person assessing you to reach an accurate conclusion about what's wrong with you, including any collateral problems that you may not have known to watch out for.

Don't feel, however, that you can't go beyond the scope of the questions asked. When it comes to diagnosis, more detail is usually better. For example, if the question is, "Have you ever experienced this type of chest pain before?" and your answer is "no," you might want to add, "I haven't felt this particular type of pain before now, but for the last few days I've been feeling kind of a tightness across the chest sometimes, and a few times it's happened, I've also had some shortness of breath."

In cases where diagnosis is difficult, it's important to be as specific as you can be about when the symptoms started. Bring up anything unusual in your routine that may be linked to your symptoms (for example, if you've eaten some new food, or the pain began not long after your return from vacation on a tropical island). Medicine is often a lot like detective work; the clues need to be noticed and pieced together to solve the problem. In this case, you're not the suspect— the disease is, and you want it caught and stopped just as much as the investigators do. (More, in fact!) To help the investigation identify the right culprit, you must do your best to answer the questions candidlyand thoroughly—even ones that strike you as irrelevant or intrusive on your personal life. Now's not the time to be coy. Besides, ER workers have seen it all and heard it all. Your story won't shock anyone, no matter what it is.

---

*Several years ago,* a landscape architect in Washington, D.C. fell from a ladder three stories high. He thought he was lucky because it seemed he'd escaped with only a broken arm. Then, several weeks later, he had an overwhelmingly severe headache. He didn't recognize it as a warning sign of anything serious and he didn't connect the headache to his fall. If he'd known to go to the emergency room, a triage nurse would have put the two things together. During the screening process he would have been asked if he had suffered any sort of head trauma within the past few weeks. A "yes" to that question would have had him sent to radiology for a CT scan. The test would have revealed that he had a subdural hematoma, a blood clot on the brain. Instead, he died.

---

**If your symptoms have changed since your arrival at the ER, make sure you report how severe they were at their worst.**
Sometimes patients who really are in bad shape appear fairly normal by the time they get to the emergency room. If the patient had a high fever but has taken aspirin or Tylenol, the ER staff would have no way of knowing how sick the patient was, unless the patient remembered to note what his temperature was at its highest point. The same is true for pain. When you're in agony, you'll do almost anything to feel better. You might dose yourself up on whatever old prescription pain medications you may have found lying around the house. You still know your pain indicates an emergency, and so you get yourself to the ER, but as the doctor pokes you here and there and asks, "How much does this hurt?" your truthful response is, "Not so much now."

This is one situation in which mistakes can be made. That's just what happened to Bill, whose story is in the box on page 192. To avoid the same fate, be sure you make your ER doctor aware of anything you may have done that would affect, and possibly alleviate, the symptoms of your condition or mislead the doctor about the diagnosis.

*Bill had had a fever* for more than a week. At first he thought it was the flu. He also had symptoms of abdominal distress: pain and diarrhea. That, too, could be part of the flu. So he stayed home, rested, drank plenty of fluids, and took fever reducers and pain pills. As the days went by, however, he realized he wasn't getting any better. One evening the pain in his stomach changed from being dull and constant to being sharp and stabbing. He called his doctor, who advised him to go to the emergency room. Right before he left the house, Bill took a narcotic painkiller; he'd already taken two Tylenols a few hours before that.

It didn't take Bill long to get to the ER, but it was more than an hour before he was seen by anyone. In that time the narcotic began to work, both dulling and diffusing the pain he was feeling. The Tylenol brought his fever down so that it was only a degree or so above normal. Bill did mention that his fever had been higher, and that he'd had it for a while, but he wasn't really sure what was the highest point because he'd been using Tylenol right from the start. Then the doctor starting moving his fingers around Bill's abdomen in a slow circle, asking him to rate the pain from 1 to 10 at each spot. "It's not so bad anymore," Bill reported truthfully. Being a relatively stoic sort of person, he was loath to complain about how horrible the pain had been an hour or so before. He did mention the pills he'd taken, but not having seen him before they took effect, the ER staff saw only a relatively healthy young man with a low fever and an upset stomach.

"Go home," the ER doctor advised him. "It's probably some kind of food poisoning. A ten-day course of antibiotics is all you need." Bill took the first pill in the hospital and went home, feeling relieved. He felt well enough to get his first good night's sleep since the illness began.

But the moment he woke up the next morning, he knew things were not good. The pain was back, far worse than it had ever been. His temperature was now 105 degrees. He felt he was in danger of losing consciousness any moment. This time he didn't stop to call his doctor. His wife drove him directly to the emergency room, where, within the hour, surgeons performed the exploratory surgery that found four perforations in his large intestine.

"It's too bad you didn't get to the hospital earlier," one of the surgeons later told him. "If your peritonitis had been treated earlier, these perforations could have been prevented."

"Actually, I *was* here earlier—I was here last night," Bill pointed out, "but my symptoms seemed mild then, so I was sent home."

### Know what to do if you're not getting the response you know you need.

You didn't come to the emergency room to wait and wait. But if it's busy and your case isn't critical, that's just what you may end up doing—maybe for hours on end. In this situation, there are three logical courses of action available:

1. You can sit and wait patiently, trusting the ER staff to get to you when the more urgent cases have been taken care of.
2. You can go back to the triage nurse and be more forceful about your need for treatment, using terms you know will prompt a speedy response.
3. You can leave the ER, either to seek treatment elsewhere, or conclude you don't have a true emergency and wait until your doctor's regular business hours to seek treatment.

If you exercise the first option, you don't need to know anything further, but if you're interested in options two and three, be sure to read the following tips.

**Restate your problem in a way that will make its urgency clear.**
To get the immediate response you need, tell the ER staff:

- "I'm having trouble breathing."
- "The pain is intense." (Be as specific as you can be about the worst spot.)
- "I feel I might lose consciousness." (Also, bring to the staff's attention any dizziness, blurred vision, sense of disorientation, or difficulty remembering where you are or what's going on around you.)
- "I can no longer move my head or neck fully." (If you are losing or have lost control over these or any other body parts, tell the nurse right away.)

If your symptoms have worsened to the point at which you can no longer say what's wrong, then you want the person accompanying you to be willing to step forward and insist that you receive prompt attention. Shyness is one trait to leave behind whenever you find yourself in the ER. But when someone you love needs you to speak up for them, even the shyest among us may find it possible to be bold. For an example, see Maggie's story in the box below.

---

*Maggie accompanied her husband* Bill to the ER. (Yes, it's the same Bill as in the story on page 192.) That morning he had woken up in extreme pain. Although he'd been to the ER the night before, the severity of his condition had gone unrecognized—his pain and other symptoms dismissed as insignificant. Now, with his condition worse than ever, both Bill and Maggie knew the situation was dire.

They arrived at the ER to find another patient with a highly unusual condition, claiming the attention of most of the staff. An assistant zookeeper had been bitten deeply by a rare type of South American monkey. The doctors were waiting to hear back

---

from experts in both tropical and veterinary medicine about the sort of diseases to take preventive measures against. Maggie heard all this recounted over the phone in the waiting room by another zoo worker who had witnessed the attack. The only other person in the room was the nurse sitting behind the reception desk, who had told Maggie and Bill upon entering to take a seat and wait.

Minutes ticked by, and the nurse didn't move from her desk. Bill continued to sit patiently, but Maggie could tell he was in agony—he was just too stoic to scream or moan. Maggie knew she couldn't let him go on that way indefinitely, and so, despite her natural shyness, she approached the nurse and said, "My husband really can't wait any longer. He's never been in pain like this before. Isn't there anyone who can see him now? I wouldn't ask unless I was sure it was necessary."

The nurse said nothing but got up to speak to someone. Within a minute, another nurse came out and called Bill's name. He was taken into a curtained-off area, where an ER doctor began the examination that, within a few more minutes, led to a surgical consult. In less than an hour Bill was being prepared for exploratory surgery to find the source of the pain. It turned out that a section of his large intestine had perforated in four places, destroyed by toxins created by a particularly virulent strain of salmonella.

Afterward, the surgeon told Bill and Maggie that if he'd waited much longer for the surgery, he would have died.

**Know who the members of the emergency care team are and what each one is there to do for you.**
When you understand "Who's Who in the Emergency Room," you won't waste time asking Nurse X for drug Y when only Doctor Z is authorized to prescribe that treatment. What follows is a brief description of some of the people you are most likely to meet either on your way to or inside the emergency room.

**Emergency medical technicians (EMTs) or paramedics.** These are the people who arrive on the scene after you call 911 or direct-dial an ambulance service. They provide certain types of urgent care (for example, CPR if your heart has stopped, oxygen if you need it, or compression and bandaging if you have a bleeding wound) and then transport you to the hospital ASAP for treatment. You should think of them as the life-and-death squad.

**Triage nurse.** Earlier in this chapter, I explained the concept of triage, sorting emergency patients into categories based on urgency of need. Some of the tips in this chapter concern how to communicate your medical needs effectively. You also want to make sure you are communicating with the right person. To be sure you're not telling your tale to a student nurse or a nurse's aide, it's a good idea to ask directly, "Are you the triage nurse?"

**Emergency room physician.** Once you make it to the doctor, the question remains, "Who is that doctor?" Many possibilities exist. It could be an emergency medicine specialist, who does nothing but deal with urgent care cases and who did residency training in emergency medicine. Or it could be a *"moonlighter,"* that is, a doctor who has a day job and is just working a few extra hours in the emergency room for added pay. That person could be an internist, a family practitioner, or maybe even a psychiatrist—any kind of specialist. Depending on the hospital's employment needs, it could be *any* medically licensed physician.

The next question is, "How do you know?" Well, unless you stop to interrogate the doctor about his résumé and experience (and few emergency room patients care to do so), you probably won't find out. However, if you've come to an ER at a big city hospital, odds are good that your case will be in the hands of (or at least overseen by) a board-certified emergency room physician. On the other hand, if you've come to the ER of a small-town hospital, that would be less likely. While the trend in ERs these days is toward staffing with specialists in emergency medicine, small-town hospitals are still experiencing too many recruiting difficulties for patients to be able to expect specialized care.

It's reassuring to learn that your ER doctor is a specialist, but I discovered from personal experience that a non-specialist can do just fine. The box below tells my story.

***

*A few years ago,* I was talking on the phone one afternoon when I had what appeared to be a mini-stroke: The side of my face drooped and I became confused. My wife rushed me to a nearby university hospital, where I was seen by a young woman who happened to be the resident on emergency room duty. After examining me and seeing that I was otherwise in good health and had now returned to normal, and after hearing about my history of migraine headaches, she concluded that what had happened to me was most likely was a manifestation of migraine. She sent me to get a CT scan. It came back normal, which ruled out any tumor, acute stroke, or mass of any kind. In this case, the episode confirmed her diagnosis that I had experienced a *migraine equivalent.* (A migraine can come not only in the form of headache, but also in the form of other symptoms and signs. It can mimic a stroke, it can mimic severe abdominal pain, and much more. Fortunately, the young doctor knew all this!) This is a good example of something that appeared to be serious—important enough to get me kicked to the top of the ER waiting list—that a doctor's keen judgment plus the right test proved to be relatively minor.

***

### Answer any and all questions from ER staff or EMTs fully, accurately, and candidly.

I've already discussed the importance of using the right words to get the attention you need. Let me also stress, as I have in other chapters of this book, the importance of revealing all possible relevant facts, even embarrassing ones. If your accident occurred because of your alcohol use or if you're there because you overdosed on an illegal drug, you've got to come out with it. Be assured that the code of doctor-patient confidentiality applies to EMTs and other emergency workers, too. Your only protection from drug interactions is to let emergency room staff know exactly what substances you have in you, in what quantity, and when you took them. Because many drug combinations can be fatal, this really is a life-and-death question.

**Follow the EMTs' instructions exactly and without argument.** Don't second-guess them about how you should be moved. The example in the box on page 199 tells how a woman almost made the fatal mistake of rejecting a neck brace. Don't argue about having your clothing cut away. Your clothes can be replaced, but body parts aren't that easy to come by. And be aware that in most jurisdictions, once the EMTs are on the scene, they are required by law to follow through with a ride to the hospital. You can't just announce that you've changed your mind and no longer want to go. Once you're at the hospital, you are free to reject any medical care you think is unnecessary—though if your condition was serious enough to warrant calling for emergency transport in the first place, you're almost certainly better off letting the emergency room doctors call the next move.

**Keep a well-stocked first aid kit in your home and in your car.** In many emergencies there are lifesaving measures you can start, well before the EMTs arrive. You may need to create a tourniquet to stop a wound from spurting blood, or use tweezers that have been cleaned with an antiseptic to remove a foreign object from your skin. In case of poisoning, you may be directed by the poison control center to use syrup of ipecac to induce vomiting. All the items named and much more should be found in your first aid kit, which you should keep in an accessible, dry storage space that does not get too hot or too cold. Rather than listing all the supplies your kit should contain, I suggest that you visit the web site of the National Library of Medicine (part of the National Institutes of Health) at: *www.nlm.nih.gov/medlineplus/firstaidemergencies.html#generaloverviews*. To get to the list of supplies to have on hand at home, click on the underlined link Your Home First Aid Kit. To see the list of supplies to keep in your car, click on the underlined link to Traveler's First Aid Kit.

> *A California skydiver* was slammed into the ground by a violent crosswind. While she was unconscious, someone dialed 911. EMTs arrived promptly and put her in a neck brace. The instant she woke up, she insisted that they remove it. She felt fine, she insisted arrogantly, and she didn't need their help. The EMTs then found themselves having to switch their efforts from treating her to calming her and restraining her from undoing their medical efforts. Given the nature of her neck injury, they knew she was at high risk of paralysis. Fortunately for her, they prevailed, and the skydiver ended up with no lasting disability (even though it appeared that her pride suffered some bangs and bumps).

Once you've bought or put together your first aid kits, remember to check them periodically, because medications expire and even well-sealed packets of antiseptic can dry out over the years. Replace and replenish them as necessary.

**Carry a cell phone and keep it turned on whenever you go out.** The terrorist attack of September 11, 2001, demonstrated what a powerful tool a cell phone can be in an emergency. Because they had cell phones, the passengers on United Airlines Flight #93 were able to call out and let the world know they were being hijacked. They were able to learn that the hijackers intended to turn their plane into a missile to destroy hundreds or even thousands more innocent lives. Although they were not able to save themselves, by acting on the knowledge they gained by using their cell phones, they were able to prevent even greater death and destruction.

Cell phones are not just for extraordinary events; they're used to bring people vital information and aid in rescues thousands of times every day. People routinely report car accidents as soon as they witness the crash; they call ambulances to their homes during storms when the normal telephone lines are down; in some cases they've brought police to a crime scene before the criminal has had a chance to escape.

(In one famous case, the victim of a carjacking was thrown into the trunk, from which she was able to dial the police surreptitiously and report her changing location as the carjacker sped down the highway. Because of her information, the police were able to set up a road-block and capture the criminal before anyone was injured or killed.)

Cell phones also allow police and emergency crews to locate acci-dent victims who can't dial out. Those few victims of the terrorist attack on the World Trade Center who were found alive were located by search crews who called their cell phone numbers and listened for the ringing amid the rubble.

So don't just carry your cell phone with you—always keep it turned on so that others can call you. (If you don't want your friends calling up to chit-chat, then don't give your number out to anyone but trusted members of your family and your designated emergency con-tact, and of course, keep your ringer turned off when you're in a res-taurant or theater.)

Cell phones are such effective emergency tools, I consider them as important as taking a CPR course or keeping a well-stocked first aid kit in your home and car. There are low-cost monthly plans that make having a cell phone affordable for almost anyone these days. And isn't your safety and your family's safety worth twenty or so dollars a month?

**Before you travel, either domestically or outside the United States, know how your insurance company will cover you in an emergency.**
Within the United States you may be required to find an emergency room that's part of your insurance plan's nationwide network. You don't want to rack up a five thousand dollar bill, only to learn that it's all out-of-pocket because you were admitted to the wrong ER for your network in that region. In case you become sick or injured out-side the United States, you'll want to find out what arrangements you can make to be flown home for treatment. Most health insurance companies do not provide for overseas air arrangements; however, you can buy a separate, overseas travel insurance policy that includes this benefit. The travel policy would cover putting you on a jet with

intensive care facilities. I would strongly urge anyone who will be visiting a country with less than first-rate medical facilities to purchase this sort of coverage as a safeguard. Any good, full service insurance agent should be able to look into your coverage options for you.

### Once you're stable in the emergency room, get in touch with a friend or relative who will take care of necessary details for you.

Someone's got to call the school and tell your child to go to the after-school program instead of expecting you to be there at pick-up time (or call your child's friend's parents and ask them to take your child home). Someone must explain to your boss why you're not coming in today. Someone must walk your dog and pick up the packages on your doorstep before the arrival of the thunderstorm that's been predicted for later in the day. It's always good to have one person on tap, who stands ready to step in for you in just such circumstances. Call that person as soon as you can, and go over the task list of what needs to be done.

Everyone needs to have someone willing to play this role for them, plus a backup if the first choice isn't available. Your emergency information card should list the person's name and contact telephone numbers (day, evening, and cell phone) so that if you can't speak, the ER nurse can make the call on your behalf.

Appendix A shows what your sample emergency card should look like.

### Ask a nurse to put your things in a safe place for you.

When you are rushed into the emergency room, the last thing you should be thinking about is your belongings—but that doesn't mean you won't be anxious about them later on. Of course, the focus at first is going to be on your medical condition—that's what you want from any emergency room staff member. But if all goes well with your treatment, you'll soon be back to more mundane concerns, and chief among them will be "What did they do with my briefcase?" You'll think to yourself, "All the notes for that presentation I've been preparing for the last three months are in there! I've got to have them!"

If you had the presence of mind at the time of your admission to request that someone keep track of your things and put them in a safe place, you'll be in good shape. If you weren't in shape to make such a request at the time, then you may discover an unfortunate truth about many big city hospital emergency rooms, which is this: Once you have been separated from your watch, jewelry, or other valuables, you just may never see them again.

If luck is with you, though, you may find yourself in a hospital with procedures in place calling for staff to set aside a patient's possessions, appropriately tagged and locked up securely until the patient is ready to have them returned. The story in the box below is a case in point.

---

***Christine, a successful*** photographer, had a traumatic motor vehicle accident in which she lost a foot. After she was stabilized at the hospital, she desperately wanted to know what happened to the possessions that had been taken from the scene of the accident: "I begged nurses to tell me where my camera equipment was. Where was my case with film in it? No one paid much attention to my questions. Their attention was totally on my injuries—I understand that. But I also felt traumatized by not knowing where my camera and film were." A friend of Christine's who was also a nurse understood both the practical reason for her question and her underlying psychological need, as a professional photographer, to know if she still had the precious camera that was almost a part of her. The nurse used her collegial influence with the nurses on duty at the time of Christine's admission to track down her friend's possessions and then bring them to her room. Christine remembers how much she was comforted by the nurse's actions, and she goes on to recommend that no one take such patient requests lightly. She says from her own experience that knowing your things have been kept safe for you can restore a sense of control and dignity that can all too easily be lost in the chaos of the emergency.

---

**Don't expect to see a real-life version of the TV show ER.**
There's usually more action in single episode of *ER* than most emergency rooms see in a week. On the TV show the same doctor who conducts the initial exam nearly always goes on to perform the operation that saves the patient's life. That's not the way it is in most real emergency rooms. In real life, ER doctors assess your condition and then decide whether to do one of three things: admit you for treatment, hang onto you for a while and observe your condition before making a treatment decision, or discharge you, with instructions for follow-up care at a non-emergency facility (if needed). If you have a private doctor and your condition isn't dire, it would be unusual for the ER doctors to initiate treatment without at least making an attempt to get in touch with your own doctor.

If you're admitted, in all but the most extreme emergencies, you'll be sent on to some other department. If it's heart symptoms, you'll be moved to the coronary care unit; if it's an infection, you'll go to the infectious disease department. Whatever your problem, the appropriate care team will be assembled to deal with it. Unlike the doctors on TV, in real life, ER doctors don't careen wildly from crisis to crisis, operating to remove a bullet from a gunshot victim one minute, then delivering a baby a few minutes later, and after that, using a defibrillator on a heart attack victim. Real life is far more boring—but that's better for you. Nobody could ever function effectively at the fever pitch of the TV drama.

Nor do you want your real-life ER doctor to be the sort of all-purpose miracle worker you see on TV, who handles everything himself, from pediatric surgery to managing AIDS. It's to your benefit when your real-life ER doctor decides not to be the one to stitch up that deep cut on your hand but calls for a consult with a plastic surgeon or a hand surgeon instead. (For an amusing look at chitchat between ER doctors, see Appendix C, "Hospital Jargon: A Sample Dialog.")

# CHAPTER 10

# Working the System to Get What You Need

This chapter is really a "who's who" of hospital personnel and a "what do they do?" for some of the more specialized workers in the hospital. When you know who's the right person to answer your question about your forthcoming MRI, you get the answer you need sooner and have a better chance to respond effectively to the information you receive. If you don't get a helpful answer from the person you've asked, then you'll know who's higher up in the chain of command to go to with your problem.

Keep in mind that the system may run a bit differently from hospital to hospital and that certain types of hospitals will have key players who aren't present in others. This chapter focuses on a typical teaching hospital, in which you find medical students and interns, who would not be present, for example, in the typical small community hospital.

### Know the players in a teaching hospital.

A teaching hospital doesn't have to be the medical center near a university campus. In the United States, university hospitals have interns, residents, fellows, and medical students, all of whom can complete a portion of their training in any community, private, or Veteran's Affairs hospital that forms an affiliation with the medical school. The new school year for all those working in university-run medical education programs begins on July 1. (See the very first tip in this book for the significance of that fact in your hospital care.)

Whether you go to a university hospital or one that participates in training of medical school students, interns, residents and fellows, you will encounter some or all of the types described in the paragraphs below. The examples appear in order from the least to the most advanced in the practice of medicine. Tips for working with doctors in training follow immediately after.

*Third and fourth year medical students* occupy the bottom rung of the authority ladder; their badges should state clearly that they are students, for example, "Joe Doe, Medical Student." A doctor on staff supervises them, but that person isn't necessarily in the room when a medical student comes to see you. They may be alone when they draw blood or ask you questions; when they're performing tests or examinations, however, a doctor will be at their side. In the operating room, given the greater ramifications if errors are made, medical students are under considerable restraint—your private surgeon and hospital staff doctors continuously supervise them. In return for the privilege of attending your operation, medical students are delegated simple, mundane tasks such as retractor holding, suture snipping, and wound stapling.

If you're going to have your operation at a university hospital, expect to have substantial contact with medical students. By the time you encounter medical students on the surgical wards, they will have completed one or two years of basic science studies in medicine, most of which were conducted in lecture halls and laboratories; they will have seen pictures in books and videos of a range of problems, from the ordinary to the bizarre. Seeing a very unusual condition on a live patient, however, is likely to captivate them in a way that you, as a patient, may find discomfiting. In short, medical students, however conscientious and enthusiastic, have limited experience in patient care.

*Interns* are a step above medical students; they are in their first year of training after medical school. An intern's badge will say, for example, "Jean Doe, PGY 1," meaning post-graduate year one, or "JAR" meaning junior assistant resident. This person has earned the degree of medical doctor but has not yet passed the professional exams or "boards" to get a license. In other words, an intern is a doctor who can only practice medicine under the supervision of a licensed physician.

In the hospital, interns rotate through different departments; the "classic five" are internal medicine, general surgery, obstetrics/gynecology, psychiatry, and pediatrics. Electives may include radiology, nuclear medicine, anesthesia—basically, any specialty or subspecialty. In July (see the discussion of the July syndrome at the beginning of Chapter 1), the new surgical interns are just learning their way around the hospital, and being called "doctor" is new to them. It will take them a few months to get comfortable with their duties on the hospital wards and, depending on the surgical training program, up to a year to be able to assist private surgeons in the operating room. Most of the surgical intern's time is spent doing the busy work that keeps them on their feet for up to 40 hours at a time. Their work involves: admitting patients; performing diagnostic procedures; checking laboratory results; drawing blood; assisting at surgery; checking your surgical wound; changing your dressing; performing a spinal tap; starting an IV catheter, central IV line, or arterial line; placing a naso-gastric tube through your nose and into your stomach; helping to supervise medical students; and doing a lot of other things that the more senior members of the hospital staff don't want to do. So when you come across an exhausted, disheveled doctor in the middle of the night, the odds are good that he or she is the intern assigned to your case.

*Residents* are a step above interns. They are doctors starting their formal training in specialties such as internal medicine, anesthesiology, obstetrics, or any of several dozen others. The resident is the person in authority when your attending surgeon or primary care physician is absent from the hospital. The residency years—designation PGY II to V—form the bulk of the graduate doctor's training. This is a time of increasing responsibility, knowledge, and development of medical skills.

Among the residents is the *chief surgical resident*—a resident in the final year of surgical training—who is the responsible person when your private surgeon is absent from the hospital. That doctor will conduct rounds, supervise medical students and interns, and report your progress to your private surgeon. Whenever a student or an intern has difficulty in performing a procedure or handling any aspect of your care, the resident is the next in line to step in to deal with the problem.

*Fellows* are in post-residency training. They are doctors who are exploring an advanced subspecialty, such as cardiology, gastro-enterology, or infectious disease. Physicians who have completed surgical residency, for example, and wish to become subspecialty surgeons (heart surgeons, cancer surgeons, colo-rectal surgeons, for example) become fellows in a department of surgery. Their designation is PGY VI to VII and beyond. By the time subspecialty surgeons complete their training, they will have spent 15 to 17 years preparing for their careers.

Attending *senior physicians* are the top doctors in charge of all these other doctors.

When it comes to decision making in your own case, it's your own *private doctor* who's the boss.

Finally, and most importantly—because you are the one who hired (and can fire) your private doctor—*you* are the ultimate person in charge of what happens to your body. Unless you are deemed incompetent, nothing can be done to you without your consent.

### When you're examined by an unfamiliar person, check his or her badge and ask questions.

Don't be intimidated by the parade of people in white coats. It's one of your basic rights as a patient to be kept informed about who is supposed to do what to you. If the doctors are properly trained in "bedside manner," they will introduce themselves before going to work on you. If anyone skips this step, call a halt so that you can check the person out. Ask bluntly, "Who are you, and why are you here?" If you don't get an answer that makes sense to you, ask your patient advocate to look into the matter for you. (See Chapter 5, page 95, for advice about choosing a patient advocate.) *Never* follow any instructions given to you in the hospital by an unknown person—the story in the box that follows tells why.

---

***Before having prostate surgery,*** Clyde asked his doctor, "What do I have to do to get out of here fast?" The doctor told him the criteria, which included things like "having a normal temperature" and "being able to walk unassisted." Clyde, very eager to go home as quickly as possible, double-checked the discharge necessities: "If I can do these things, then you'll let me out—right?" The doctor said, "Sure." After the four-hour surgery, Clyde began to tackle the conditions for his release one by one. He sat up. Then, as soon as he was able to walk, he "did a dance past the nurses' station once an hour," as he described it to me.

The next morning, a "guy in a white uniform" popped into Clyde's room and said, "Is there anything I can do for you?"

Clyde said, "I want to take a shower."

The nice young man was very accommodating: "I'll set it up for you."

So Clyde wheeled his IV stand into the shower, which is where a shocked nurse found him soaping down.

"What are you doing? You can't take a shower!" she gasped. By then, all of Clyde's dressings were falling off. It took the nurse two hours to redo them. Clyde was banned from going anywhere until the new dressings could be checked. That brought an end to his dance past the nurses' station and his hopes of setting a new record for release from the hospital after prostate surgery.

And the nice young man in the white coat? Clyde never saw him again, and no one seemed to know who he was.

---

**If you're bothered by too many visits from doctors in training, ask your private doctor or the attending senior doctor to take matters in hand.**

In certain complicated cases it's of benefit to you to have more doctors involved in your treatment and watching out for complications. Most of the time, though, the benefit is primarily one-way: Your case provides the doctor in training with material to study. If the teaching hospital is efficiently run, then procedures will be in place to minimize redundant exams and unnecessary intrusions. You'll just have more people observing during visits that would have occurred in any case. But if the system is not so well coordinated, the interruptions and repetitions can really get out of hand. It doesn't have to be that way. You have only to ask to protect yourself from turning into the learning experience for too many doctors in training, as Lena found out in the story below.

***When Lena slipped*** on an icy sidewalk, she suffered a severe fracture to her hip and was rushed to a major teaching hospital. Only 39 years old, she suddenly faced the nightmare of many elderly patients—a total hip replacement. Four doctors examined her in the emergency room. "Which one is really responsible for me?" she wondered in a panic.

After her emergency surgery, she recalls, "It was impossible to get more than three hours of sleep at night. I was constantly being awakened by doctors and students." Each morning at about four o'clock, she would open her eyes to the aggravating sight of eight to ten doctors and students standing by her bedside, reviewing her chart, examining her, mumbling to each other, and asking her how she felt. "How do most people feel at four o'clock in the morning?" she snapped.

Finally, Lena asked the nurses and her attending doctor to allow only essential personnel into her room. That's all she had to do! They met her request immediately, and for the first time since her injury, she got a good night's sleep.

## Don't allow anyone with shaky skills to perform procedures on you.

There's no reason you must let a medical student learn the necessary skills on you. If you're approached by a medical student in a manner that suggests the person is less than confident and experienced at the job at hand, don't hesitate to say, "Wait! I'd like a nurse to do that" (draw blood, change a dressing, or whatever). If you're not sure whether the student has sufficient experience to be competent, then come right out and ask, "How long have you been doing this?"—and don't accept a vague answer like, "Oh, for a while now." You want the response to be something along the lines of "I've done it hundreds of times," or, at the very least, "dozens of times." Don't worry about how the poor medical student is supposed to find someone willing to be provide one of the first dozen learning experiences—that's not your problem. (It's most likely the problem of the patient in the next room who was never cautioned to ask questions and take self-protective actions while in the hospital, as you have been now.)

## Consider the benefits of medical student involvement.

Because students are in a period of intense academic growth, and because they have more free time than the hospital staff doctors, you'll find them more meticulous in their questioning and performance of physical examinations. They may even tire you out with their thoroughness. In some cases, that can be a good thing. Any experienced doctor (if not too arrogant to admit it) can tell you about a case in which he or she missed some important physical finding that had bearing on the patient's outcome, only to have it pointed out by an attentive medical student. The box on page 212 is a story that comes from my own experience.

## Consider the intern assigned to your case a good source of reliable information about your progress.

Because of a high caseload, your private surgeon may not have the time to sit with you and address every question and concern you have. Your intern is far more likely to be willing to play this role. Ask him or her to get answers to the things you want to know: How long until

> **When I was a resident,** a woman came to the outpatient surgical center where I worked to have an extensive oral surgery. Before getting started, an intern performed a cursory physical examination and found nothing unusual. A medical student, on the other hand, noticed a heart murmur. He asked the intern to listen again.
>
> Eventually, the diagnosis of mitral valve prolapse was made, and the patient received prophylactic (preventive) antibiotics before her surgery. If the student hadn't been present, the heart murmur and the condition it indicated would have gone unnoticed and untreated. The surgery might well have resulted in a mitral valve infection—a serious problem that's not always easy to treat.

you can get out of bed? What did the pathology report reveal? When can the tubes be removed? These issues are discussed in rounds every day, and it is part of the intern's job to help find the right solutions to your needs. Your intern is also the person to ask about the hours of rounds (see the next tip).

### Know the schedule of rounds.

You've seen them at odd hours, roaming the hospital corridors—a gaggle of doctors, trailed by an assortment of interns, residents, fellows, and other members of the hospital staff (collectively known as *house staff*). They wander from room to room, from bed to bed, usually at ungodly hours of the morning. These wanderings are called *rounds,* and it is on rounds that these medical nomads discuss, in practical and theoretical terms, every aspect of each patient's case.

You may not like being awakened early in the morning for rounds, but you may find it easier to cope with the wake-up once you are fully briefed on when rounds occur and whom to expect to see. The intern assigned to your case is the most accessible source of information about the rounds that involve you.

## Know who is an M.D. and who is a D.O., and understand the difference.

House staff, that is, hospital staff doctors, may be either one—but they're not the same. An M.D. has earned the doctor of medicine degree after completing four years of medical school, and before that, having earned a Bachelor of Science or Arts degree at a four-year college (although there are a few medical school that award the M.D. degree to students who complete a combined six-year undergraduate/ medical program). A D.O. (doctor of osteopathy) has graduated from a school of osteopathy, which may or may not require that its students be college graduates (although these days, most are). Osteopathic schools are founded upon the philosophy of Andrew Taylor Still (1828-1917), who believed that most diseases are caused by mechanical interference with the nerves and blood supply and are curable by manipulation of "deranged, displaced bones, nerves, and muscles— removing all obstructions—thereby setting the machinery of life moving." He called his treatment method "osteopathic manipulative treatment" (OMT) and sought to have it used in place of traditional approaches using drugs and surgery. In modern osteopathic schools, OMT is no longer taught as a replacement for all other methods; it's taught in addition to practices involving drugs and surgery.

To learn more about the differences in education and medical philosophy between M.D.s and D.O.s you might want to read the very detailed report found on the Quackwatch website at *www. quackwatch.com/04ConsumerEducation/QA/osteo.html*.

## Rely on house staff at times when your private doctor is unavailable.

Because surgical house staff practically live in the hospital, they're even more likely to be attuned to your immediate medical needs than your own surgeon. It will be the house staff doctor who follows a falling hematocrit (red blood cell count) over the course of sixteen hours and informs your surgeon of the need to operate, even though it is your surgeon who makes the actual decision to operate. When you're home at three o'clock in the morning and you suddenly wake up with a sharp, twisting pain in your belly, your private doctor may send you to the emergency room to be evaluated by house staff doctors. In most cases, all the necessary laboratory tests and physical findings will be recorded in your chart by the time your surgeon arrives. Think of house staff as the doctors on the front lines and your private surgeon as the field commander responsible for making the final decisions.

### If you're having a problem the intern can't seem to handle, get the resident involved.

The resident has authority when your surgeon or physician is absent from the hospital. If the matter isn't so urgent as to require a call to your private doctor's emergency number, then the resident is the person you want looking into things for you.

### Don't let communication problems persist between you and house staff doctors.

One of the first things you may notice when you meet house staff, especially if you are in a big city hospital, is that many of the doctors come from other countries. While it's good that American hospitals are able to recruit the best and the brightest from all over the world, there can be disadvantages, too, especially if the hospital does not check before hiring to be sure that the doctor is fully conversant in colloquial American English. You want to be sure you are clear on the doctor's instructions, and equally sure, when you explain your problem or report your symptoms, that you have been understood.

If you find yourself continually asking the same doctor to repeat or restate something, or if you've said something to a doctor that has either left the doctor staring blankly at you or elicited the wrong response, then you're in a situation calling for help from someone higher up in the hospital chain of command. Inform the supervising doctor or your own doctor of the problem with communication. Give specific examples of any miscommunication that has occurred. There are two possible solutions: Either make sure that a fluent speaker of English is on hand whenever you're communicating with the doctor, to verify that correct information is flowing in both directions, or ask that the doctor who's ineffective at communicating with you be taken off your case.

## Don't accept rudeness or dismissive behavior from house staff doctors.

Just because someone is a hospital doctor doesn't mean that everything he or she does is allowed in that hospital. No one should be permitted to call a patient names, disregard real medical needs, or treat appropriate requests with contempt. You can complain to your own doctor or the attending senior physician—or if the offending doctor is an intern or resident, complain to the chief resident—or all three. If you're not in shape to complain on your own, your patient advocate should lodge the complaint for you. In well-run hospitals, supervisors want to hear if any doctors are not living up to the highest professional standards. Your complaint won't be just filed and forgotten.

At the same time, patients need to keep in mind that being a resident or an intern is a tough job, often exhausting, and more often than not, patience trying. Young doctors in training are routinely treated harshly themselves: Patients scream at them, older doctors scold them for errors, and nurses get annoyed at their inexperience. It's always worthwhile to try a gentle approach first: "I know you didn't mean to snap at me just now when I asked you to repeat your question. You may have forgotten that it's my left ear that's affected. You need to stand to my right for me to hear you better." If that doesn't get you an apology before the doctor repeats the question, then you know that the person isn't just having an off day; he's probably rude all the time—and you're right to complain about him.

## Never accept harassment of any kind from a doctor, and report any such incidents at once.

In some cases you don't want to give the doctor a second chance. There's never any excuse for inappropriately touching a patient, making sexual suggestions or advances, or using offensive language. Don't let any time pass before reporting such behavior, either. Your ability to document what happened is dependent on your accuracy with details: time, place, and exactly what was said or done by whom. The problem is what to do about ambiguous cases: For example, you're in the hospital for a gynecological problem, and so the doctor had reason to be touching your genitals, but you believe his handling of you felt more like fondling. In such an instance, you may want to express concern without making a specific charge. The best course is simply to tell the supervising physician that the doctor has made you feel uncomfortable, and request not to be alone with that doctor. Hospitals will honor such requests, if only to protect themselves from the more serious charge of failure to act to protect patients when warned.

**If there are multiple doctors involved in your treatment, make sure they check with each other before subjecting you to any procedures or major changes in your treatment.**
In Chapter 7, you'll find the story about a post-surgical patient, Addison, whose case was of interest not just to his own surgeon but also to the doctors of the hospital's infectious disease department, who were curious about the source of the food poisoning that caused the perforations in his large intestine. The department head ordered Addison brought in for a painful, invasive test to retrieve samples of the pathogen. His surgeon had neither ordered nor known about the test. It didn't occur to Addison to ask whether the doctors in one department of the hospital were coordinating his care with any of the others. Now, of course, he knows better—and so do you.

**Keep in mind, you can always go right to the top—to your doctor—when you need to.**
While it's useful to know what kind of complaints you can bring to the chief resident, the senior attending physician, or your hospital's patient advocacy office, it's not essential information. Your well-being in the hospital is your own doctor's responsibility, and so you should be able to bring complaints directly to him or her. If it's not some-thing your doctor can fix directly, then he or she should be able to tell you who can. Your doctor, is, after all, the person who admitted you to that hospital, the one who works with that hospital's staff, the one who knows the ropes. Educating yourself about the hospital system is all to the good, but you're still not likely to be as effective in calling attention to problems that need to be solved as your doctor would be. So if it's a critical issue, waste no time working your way up the

chain of command. Call in the top officer, and if you've got a good one, let him or her get the troops up to snuff.

**If you have a complicated case that has perplexed the staff at your local hospital, take advantage of the hospital's use of *telemedicine.***

Telemedicine is the use of computer, imaging, and communications equipment by hospital staff members to close the geographic gap between those who have a medical need and those who have the specialized expertise to help.

These days many hospitals, even those in small communities, are equipped to practice telemedicine, communicating with doctors around the world via a combination of fax machines, digital cameras, Internet access, and other now-standard technologies. At the Medical College of Georgia (MCG), for example, there is a program that since 1991 has connected patients from remote, underserved rural areas of the state to doctors at its affiliated hospital in Augusta. Thus, patients sitting with their family doctor in the Dodge County Hospital can have the benefit of diagnosis and treatment recommendations from specialists at the MCG, 130 miles away, saving them from both the expense and the difficulty of traveling while ill.

If your case presents unusual issues, your doctor or others on staff at the hospital may ask for your permission to communicate your test results, history, and MRI, ultrasound, or other diagnostic images over the Internet to specialists at a university hospital or research center. Telemedicine has sometimes been able to provide solutions for difficult cases that in another era would have been given up for lost.

**Know the members of the nursing and physician's assistant staff.**

More and more these days, in hospitals large and small, doctors are doing less and nurses and physician's assistants are doing more. This trend is mainly driven by the economic engine of medicine, which is fuelled by reimbursement patterns of health insurance companies: Doctors get paid a lot; nurses and physician's assistants earn far less and so are better for the company's bottom line. They may be limited in the services they provide, but for routine screening and simple treatment, in most cases, the quality of care has been found to be as good. Later in this chapter, you will find advice about when to request a doctor rather than let a nurse-practitioner or a physician's assistant handle your care.

What follows immediately are brief descriptions of some common hospital occupations: registered nurse; nurse-practitioner; physician's assistant; various other types of advanced practice nurse; licensed practical nurse; licensed vocational nurse; unlicensed assistive personnel.

*Registered nurse.* While you're in the hospital, you should expect your day-to-day care to be in the hands of registered nurses (RNs). On each shift you may have a single RN assigned to respond to your medical needs and watch out for your physical comfort. Your RN is responsible for the basics of your care, making sure your doctor's instructions are carried out, medications are delivered as ordered, and your daily progress is tracked. Nurses monitor your condition at regular intervals, note any changes on your chart, and keep doctors up to date on the information. In most hospitals RNs are the foot-soldiers of medicine—always there, working hard, slogging through the daily grind—while the "brass" (the doctors who give the orders) receive all the glory.

RNs typically enter the profession through either of two career paths: They receive a B.S.N. (bachelor of science in nursing) after completing the course requirements in a four-year nursing school or they receive an A.D.N. (associate's degree in nursing) after completing a two-year program (usually through a community college rather than a specific nursing school). In either case they must pass a state licensing examination.

RNs who go on to additional years of study and who meet higher-level licensing requirements are known as *advanced practice nurses (APNs);* among them are various types of specialized nurses, including nurse-practitioners (NPs), certified nurse midwives (CNMs), and certified registered nurse anesthetists (CRNAs), as well as many other clinical nurse specialists (CSNs), several of whom are described later in this chapter.

*Nurse-practitioner.* NPs are registered nurses who have passed advanced courses and been licensed by the state to perform many of the functions formerly restricted to physicians. NPs may: take patient histories; perform physical exams; order laboratory tests and diagnostic procedures; and manage certain types of therapies, including prescribing medications and making referrals to specialists. NPs are most often found in family practice or general medicine, but increasingly they are coming to play a role in any setting in which a physician provides care, including the operating room. Their scope of practice varies quite a bit from state to state.

The NP career path grew out of nursing, with the first nurse-practitioner educational program having been developed as a master's degree curriculum at the University of Colorado School of Nursing in 1965. These days NPs hold both a bachelor's degree and a master's degree in nursing science, and have a minimum of three years' practice as a registered nurse.

Currently, most states allow some form of third-party (insurance) reimbursement for treatment by NPs; federal law specifically authorizes Medicaid reimbursement to certified family or pediatric NPs at the same rate that doctors get paid for the same service in the local area.

*Physician's assistant.* The PA profession has its roots in the military system of medics and corpsmen. As the occupation evolved and was incorporated into civilian life, the educational requirements have become somewhat standardized, so that now a typical PA will have a minimum of two years of college (though, increasingly, the trend is toward a four-year college degree), followed by practical experience within a health care setting, for example, as an EMT or an RN, and then completion of a twenty- to twenty-four-month PA program in a college of medicine.

PAs, like NPs, perform many of the basic functions of a primary care physician. (See the NP description above for the list of skills.)

They usually work within a family medicine practice, often under the direct supervision of physicians. If that's the case, the billing will also be under the physician's name, so that there is no problem with insurance, Medicare, or Medicaid reimbursement.

For a side-by-side comparison between PAs and NPs, see the table below.

|  | **Nurse Practitioner (NP)** | **Physician's Assistant (PA)** |
|---|---|---|
| **Education** | Bachelor's degree, master's degree in nursing | Minimum of 2 years of college, although most PAs today are graduates of 4-year colleges, then completion of a 20- to 24 month program at a medical college |
| **Work experience** | Typically, 3-year minimum as an RN | PAs typically have served as military medical corps personnel, or have been EMTs or medics in some other health care setting |
| **Duties** | History taking; patient examination; diagnosis; ordering tests and procedures; managing therapy, including making referrals to specialists and prescribing drugs | History taking; patient examination; diagnosis; ordering tests and procedures; managing therapy, including making referrals to specialists and prescribing drugs |

*Clinical nurse specialist (CNS).* Depending on area of specialization and interests, you might find a CNS in any of the following roles: educator, case manager, consultant, researcher, administrator, or clinician. For example, in the neonatal intensive care unit you might find a CNS in the pediatric cardiology department, taking care of newborns with heart defects. A CNS in geriatric medicine might be the manager or even the chief executive of a nursing home for the elderly. A CNS in infectious diseases might travel from school to school, educating teens about prevention of sexually transmitted diseases.

Two different types of CNSs who are commonly found in hospitals are described below.

*Certified nurse-midwife (CNM).* CNMs provide care for women during normal pregnancy, labor, and delivery, and they also provide care for the newborn immediately after birth. Some CNMs offer routine gynecological and family planning services as well. They work in a variety of settings under different arrangements: They may come to the woman in labor to deliver her baby at home, be associated with a birthing center or maternity clinic, work in partnership with obstetricians in a hospital, or be part of a broad health care organization such as an HMO. They train and are certified according to a program approved by the American College of Nurse-Midwives.

*Certified registered nurse-anesthetist (CRNA).* CRNAs have six to eight years of nursing and anesthesia training and, in some settings, function without the oversight of anesthesiologists. In fact, CRNAs are the sole anesthesia provider in at least 65 percent of rural hospitals, according to the American Association of Nurse Anesthetists. In many hospitals the anesthesia for various types of procedures will be managed by a team composed of both doctors and CRNAs. Such an arrangement can lead to the highest quality of care, in my opinion, because the team draws upon the skills of diverse professionals trained in a broad variety of techniques. How to find out whether a nurse-anesthetist will be involved in your anesthesia care is discussed in Chapter 4, "All About Anesthesia."

*Licensed practical nurse (LPN)/Licensed vocational nurse (LVN).* There is little practical difference between LPNs and LVNs when it comes to level of education and skills. Both are trained in basic nursing duties and are employed by hospitals to provide direct patient care. Neither LPNs nor LVNs are required to have a college degree, and many take and pass the state licensing exam after having completed only a few nursing courses at a community college or vocational school. Usually a year's supervised service in a hospital is also part of the training process.

Different hospitals give their LPNs and LVNs a varying scope of duties. In some hospitals, although they are nominally lower down in the hierarchy than RNs, they are allowed to do virtually everything that the RNs do. In other hospitals they are quite limited in their functions, and are more likely to be found changing bed linens and fetching bedpans. Later in this chapter I have some advice for patients about when to insist upon the services of an RN, rather than a lower-level nurse or a nurse's aide.

*Nurse's aide; unlicensed assistive personnel.* Back in the old days (when I was in medical school), things were much more clear-cut: You had nurses, who took orders from doctors, and you had nurse's aides, who took orders from nurses. These days it's often hard to figure out who reports to whom. Many hospitals have invented new terms for different types of assistants in the system. The term "nurse's aide," once commonplace, seems to be falling out of favor. In its place is the unrevealing acronym, UAP, standing for "Unlicensed Assistive Personnel." (My word processing program keeps signaling me that there is no such word as "assistive" in the English language—but perhaps if more hospitals keep using it, it will be added.)

Whatever they're called, UAPs assist the nurse in patient care, but usually they are quite restricted in what they are allowed to do. They may have very little formal education, with employment requirements varying widely from hospital to hospital. Some UAPs are undergraduate students on their way to becoming nurses, doctors, or therapists, and so they may actually have some scientific or medical knowledge about patient care. Most, however, have drifted into the job from other minimum-wage employment—although if they're bright, observant, and ambitious, they may learn a lot as they gain experience over the years of working with nurses and other trained medical assistants.

The trouble comes when hospital administrators, in a cost-cutting move, assign hastily-trained UAPs to tasks that only RNs or, at the very least, well-trained and experienced LPNs, ought to do. Unfortunately, I believe the economics of today's health care system creates a strong incentive for hospitals to continue to expand the role of UAPs into areas that were formerly off-limits to them. Later in this chapter

I will offer some tips for ways to make sure that when you need skilled care, you receive it only from professionals who have been trained to provide it.

### Get to know your regular RNs well.
While student nurses tend to rotate among departments, RNs are usually assigned to a particular area, such as surgery, maternity, pediatrics, the emergency room, intensive care, cardiology, or other departments. That means that during your hospital stay you are likely to see the same faces at the same times of day, every day. It's to your benefit to get to know your regular RNs well, and make sure they become familiar with you. Be friendly. Ask the nurse how she's doing, inquire about her family, and tell her about yours. That way you'll become more to her than just "the kidney stone in Room 428."

### Go to your nurse with the sort of everyday problems your doctor doesn't handle.
Your doctor isn't going to be much help if your room is too hot or too cold. He isn't the one to complain to when the patient down the hall has turned the TV volume way up. Although he might be willing to prod the nurses to be more attentive to you when you feel that your overall quality of care needs improvement, he should not be involved in the minutiae of your care. Look upon your nurse as the one who knows how to deal with the day-to-day problems of hospital life.

### The nurse can be a reliable conduit to your doctor.
Sometimes a word to your nurse will get a faster response than trying to get through to the right doctor on your own. That's what Gina found out when she was in pain after cancer surgery and wanted an increase in her dose of narcotics. She wasn't sure which of the several doctors she'd seen was the one to issue the order. One by one, the doctors who checked on her told her to try someone else. She assumed she'd eventually find the right one to write the prescription that would give her relief. The one person she didn't "bother" was the nurse on duty. Later, when the nurse finally heard of her predicament, she told Gina she would have been glad to relay her request to the right

doctor, if only she'd been asked. It was part of her job, she explained, to look after her patients' needs and see to it that doctors were promptly notified when those needs weren't being met.

### If you're unhappy with your nurse, request a change.

Some nurses are pleasant and helpful. Others treat you as if you're a nuisance and your every request is a burden. Sometimes the nurse is trying to be helpful, but she may have communication problems, either because she speaks English with a heavy accent or she doesn't understand your regional or colloquial use of English. If, for whatever reason, you find a nurse unable to meet your ordinary hospital needs, don't keep quiet. You have a right to considerate and effective care. If, despite your best efforts to get the nurse to be more responsive, you still find her inadequate to the job, let the head nurse know. Be specific about each problem you have experienced. (This is also something for your patient advocate to take up.) The head nurse should take prompt action to change assignments and get you someone who will better serve your needs; however, if your complaints result in no action, appeal to the hospital's patient advocacy office or discuss the situation with your own doctor.

### If you're assigned a physician's assistant or a nurse-practitioner when you would rather have a doctor, say so.

The best time to put in the request is when you're scheduling an examination, test, or procedure. Ask, "Will I be seeing a doctor for this or a PA (or an NP)?" You may be told that your insurance plan provides for reimbursement only at the PA or NP pay scale for that particular service. (This will generally be the case if your hospital or clinic is in a largely rural area or if you belong to an HMO.) If so, and you still insist upon having a doctor instead, then be prepared to pay for the difference out of pocket.

If you don't discover until you arrive that you'll be seeing an NP or a PA, and you would prefer a doctor, you may have to reschedule. It's a good idea to find out through a little investigation ahead of time if the particular exam or procedure you're having is something normally handled by doctors or it's now become standard for patients to be sent to a PA or an NP. Although I would still prefer an M.D. for anything calling for advanced skills or judgment, I have seen that most PAs and NPs do a perfectly fine job at myriad day-to-day diagnostic and treatment tasks without a doctor's supervision. Of course, if any particular PA or NP appears to do a less than competent job, you should certainly waste no time in requesting a change.

### Know who's an RN, who's an LPN or LVN, and who isn't a nurse at all.

Nurses will usually introduce themselves by saying, "I'm [name] and I'll be your nurse this afternoon," but they seldom tell you exactly what sort of nurse they are. However, the nurse's name badge should include this information. Don't try to figure it out by color of attire: The days when all RNs dressed in white are gone, as are their distinctive caps. If you can't make out the "alphabet soup" on the badge, it's perfectly fine to ask, "Are you an RN?" Nurses who have earned the degree will be proud to tell you so, and those who haven't are forbidden from passing themselves off as such.

### Don't let an LPN or LVN do anything you can see is beyond that person's skill level.

If you find that an LPN's skills fall short in some area—a painful IV start, for example—ask an RN to take over. Don't worry about offending the nurse who has lesser skills: Worry only about protecting yourself from someone who might have been assigned a task she isn't fully competent to perform.

To avoid having to find out whether the LPN has the skills or not, you might want to let the head nurse know right from the start of your hospitalization that you want all advanced nursing duties to be carried out by RNs only. For a list of tasks considered to be advanced, see the bullet list in the next tip.

### Watch out for UAPs taking on functions that should belong only to qualified nurses or doctors.

According to a 1996 report by the Institute of Medicine (an affiliate of the National Academy of Sciences), most unlicensed aides have no more than a high school diploma, and close to 20 percent are high school dropouts. (This report was cited by writer Andrea Rock in her article "How Hospitals Are Gambling with Your Life," in the September 2001 issue of *Reader's Digest.*) Rock's article goes on to detail case after case of medical malpractice committed by untrained, unqualified UAPs thrust into hospital positions that used to be filled by nurses. In a sidebar to her article Rock strongly cautions readers against letting anyone but an RN perform any of the following services:

- inserting IVs, catheters, or gastric tubes
- changing sterile dressings or treating damaged skin
- giving shots
- caring for a tracheostomy
- giving tube feedings

Let me add, I heartily concur with her recommendations.

---

*Anne was caring* for her mother, who, after having been diagnosed with terminal cancer, expressed a desire to die at home. Anne arranged for nurses to come and administer IV drugs as needed to make her mother's final days comfortable. No one at nursing agency explained to her the difference between RNs and LPNs. Just the opposite, Anne was assured that LPNs were fully qualified to change bags of IV fluids. Because that was the only special skill involved in her mother's care (the other duties were mainly housekeeping, errand running, cooking, and bathing), Anne saw no reason to pay more to have RNs.

From the first day, however, the LPNs sent out by the agency proved unsatisfactory. One didn't even know how to put on sterile gloves: She kept trying to pull them on over the many large-stoned rings on her fingers. Another would yank on Anne's mother's IV line, once pulling so hard that she caused the needle to pop out. The night-shift LPN regularly fell asleep, not waking up even when Anne's mother cried for assistance. Not one of them spoke English with enough fluency to make themselves understood—one was not even literate enough to read the doctor's instructions.

After that disastrous first week, Anne decided to switch to RNs for all tasks related to the administration of IV drugs. The agency charged more than double the rate for an RN as for an LPN, and so Anne could no longer afford round-the-clock nursing care. But for all the unskilled tasks—the cleaning and shopping and simply having a responsible person present to call for a doctor if needed—Anne found a live-in housekeeper with a warm and caring personality. The RNs visited four times a day to perform their nursing tasks with skill and efficiency. This arrangement proved both cost effective and satisfactory until the end of Anne's mother's life.

### Beware of badges bearing vague labels.

I've warned you to read the badge, but what do you do when the badge says something like "patient care associate" or "patient care partner"? Just what does that mean? I doubt you'll get an honest answer when you ask, so I'll tell you now: It means absolutely nothing. Nobody you will ever meet—whether a nurse, a doctor, or any other sort of hospital worker—went to "patient care school." To learn something useful when only vagueness is being offered, you may need to pin down your respondent with yes-or-no questions. Ask, "Are you an RN? An LPN? Do you have any sort of license to perform medical procedures?" See the tip above for advice about the specific procedures that only an RN should perform.

### Know the various therapists and technicians who work at the hospital and what they can do for you.

The cast of characters you meet in the hospital includes far more than just doctors, nurses, students, and aides. There is an ever-expanding list of therapists and technicians, most of whom have specialized occupational names. This book does not have space for me to describe them all; the ones you'll find below are merely those most commonly found at work in various hospital departments and clinics.

(For a brief description of some of the most commonly performed hospital procedures you may find mentioned below, be sure to read Appendix B.)

*Dietitian/nutritionist.* The hospital's chief dietitian is in charge of the meal program at the hospital. A clinical dietitian or nutritionist will counsel you about the need to change your food consumption patterns after your doctor has diagnosed you with any condition that is directly impacted by your diet (such as diabetes, high cholesterol, high blood pressure, some kidney problems, obesity). Meals in the hospital should conform to your new dietary requirements. You should also be provided with resources (continued counseling sessions, meal-planning guides, cooking classes, and so forth) to enable you to stick to your new dietary regime at home for as long as your health requires it.

*Occupational therapist (OT).* OTs help people improve their ability to perform everyday tasks. If you've had a stroke, an OT would help you relearn and practice basic skills like dressing and eating; he or she might also give you exercises to improve your memory or hand-eye coordination. After a disabling accident, an OT would be the one to help you learn to use any adaptive equipment, such as a wheelchair or a walker. OTs have also been involved in rehabilitation of patients with alcoholism, drug abuse, depression, eating disorders, or stress-related disorders, teaching patients how to reorganize their daily lives around productive, achievable goals and avoid situations and behaviors that in the past have triggered the problematic response.

*Physical therapist (PT).* PTs use exercise, physical manipulation, and related therapies to help recovering heart attack and stroke victims, surgical patients, injured athletes, children with developmental problems or cerebral palsy, and others who need rehabilitation after injury or disease. (As you can see, there is considerable overlap between PTs and OTs. If you are confused about why you are seeing one rather than the other, ask the therapist to draw the distinction for you.)

*Recreational therapist.* These therapists are also known as "therapeutic recreation specialists." They usually treat patients suffering from depression, stress, or anxiety (which may or may not be the primary reason the patient has been hospitalized). Recreational therapy typically involves a patient in activities such as music, dancing, art, and/or games designed to lift the patient's spirits and energy level and restore a sense of emotional well-being.

*Respiratory therapist.* Breathe deeply. Under the direction of your physician, a respiratory therapist will evaluate, treat, and care for you if you have a breathing disorder. The respiratory therapist will have you breathe into an instrument that measures the volume and flow of air during inhalation and exhalation to test your lung capacity. He or she may also draw blood to analyze oxygen and carbon dioxide concentration. Respiratory therapists treat all types of patients, ranging from newborns whose lungs are underdeveloped to older people whose lungs have become diseased. If you are in the hospital for asthma or emphysema, or if you are receiving emergency care for heart failure, stroke, or shock, you can expect to receive respiratory therapy. Don't be alarmed if the person who connects your breathing tube to a ventilator isn't wearing a badge with the title of doctor—it's entirely appropriate for the person providing this service to be a respiratory therapist.

*Speech-language pathologist/audiologist.* If an illness or injury impairs your ability to use or process language or to hear, a speech-language pathologist or an audiologist will come to your aid. Speech-language pathologists generally work with people who can't speak normally, but they may also work with people who have oral motor problems that cause eating and swallowing difficulties. You might develop problems such as these if you have had a stroke, for example, or if you've sustained head injuries in an accident.

Audiologists focus on hearing, balance, and other ear-related problems. They use several different testing devices to determine the nature and extent of your hearing loss. Hearing disorders can result from a variety of causes, including injury, infection, genetic diseases, and aging.

*Cardiovascular technologist/technician.* You will see cardiovascular technologists and technicians in the hospital if you have a problem with your heart or blood vessels. If you go in for an angioplasty, a procedure used to treat blockages of blood vessels, a technologist would assist your doctor in inserting a catheter with a balloon on the end to the point of the obstruction. The technologist is the one who prepares you for the procedure by positioning you on the examining table, then shaving, cleaning, and in some cases, administering anesthesia to the top of the your leg where the catheter is inserted. During the procedure, the technologist monitors your blood pressure and heart rate with electrocardiogram (EKG) equipment and notifies your doctor if something looks wrong.

Some cardiovascular technologists specialize in noninvasive tests that diagnose problems with your circulation. They use ultrasound instruments to collect information about blood pressure, circulation, and heart function. You might have these tests during or immediately after surgery, and the technologists and technicians who administer in them are called *echocardiographers.*

There are many other heart-related tests that cardiovascular technicians may perform on patients, including the treadmill stress tests in which the patient walks on a treadmill while hooked up to an EKG monitor. If you've ever had this test, you'll know that the technician is the person who keeps turning up the treadmill speed another notch, when you think you can't possibly go any faster.

*Clinical laboratory technologist/technician.* Also called medical technologists and technicians, clinical laboratory technologists and technicians examine and analyze body fluids, tissues, and cells to help doctors diagnose and treat disease. The one you've undoubtedly met before is the *phlebotomist,* who takes blood samples.

*Electroneurodiagnostic technologist.* Electroneurodiagnostic technologists help physicians to diagnose a number of different brain disorders, including brain tumors, strokes, and epilepsy. Using an electroencephalograph (EEG) machine, which records electrical impulses transmitted by the brain and the nervous system, they can also measure the effects of infectious diseases on the brain. These technologists play a key role in assessing the probability of recovery from a coma and determining if brain death has occurred.

*Nuclear medicine technologist.* Nuclear medicine technologists use radioactive material to highlight a specific organ or area of the body and make an image of it. In some cases, they use a tiny needle to inject a radioactive tracer. (The process hurts as much—or as little—as having a needle inserted to draw blood.) In another test, the patient is required to swallow or inhale the radioactive material; the technologist then operates a camera that detects and maps the tracer as it travels inside the body. The result is an image on photographic film or a computer monitor that shows the concentration and distribution of the tracer.

*Radiologic technologist.* Just think "X-ray" and "MRI." Radiologic technologists use diagnostic imaging equipment to record the condition of your insides. Radiographers, commonly referred to as X-ray technicians, work with (you guessed it) X-rays. The technologist who takes images of the breasts to screen for cancer or other breast anomalies is called a *mammographer.* The box below lists some questions you might want to ask of your radiologic technologist.

---

**Some good questions for your radiologic technologist are**

- How long is this going to take? (Certain types of problems need to be imaged from many different angles.)
- What happens if I move while you're taking a picture?
- Is the MRI closed or open?
- Is the machine noisy? If so, will I be able to mask the noise by listening to music over headphones? Do you have headphones, or should I bring my own?
- Can I talk to you while this is going on?
- Can a family member be there with me or behind the shield with you?
- Do you recommend that I ask my doctor for a sedative to take beforehand?

---

*Surgical technician/technologist.* Before your operation, the surgical technologists, who are also called surgical or operating room technicians, help set up the operating room with surgical instruments and other equipment, sterile linens, and sterile solutions. It's possible that a surgical technologist, rather than an OR nurse, will be the one to wash and shave you before surgery, wheel you into the OR, help position you on the operating table, and cover you with sterile surgical drapes. During surgery, technologists may pass instruments and other sterile supplies to surgeons and surgeon assistants, and do a number of other key jobs, such as count sponges and needles to make sure nothing ends up left inside you. After your operation, surgical technologists will help get you to the recovery room and clean up the OR for the next patient.

**Ask if the dietitian will be available to monitor your progress and help you work through any problems with your diet after your discharge from the hospital.**
If the answer is no, then ask for a referral to a dietitian who sees outpatients. A change in eating habits is never a one-shot kind of

*Kristen, a 45-year-old* patient with a certification in personal training and a long history as a competitive athlete, wasn't comfortable with the physical therapy approach her doctor first recommended. After an initial pre-operative visit with the therapist, Kristen returned to her doctor to report her frustrations with what had gone on in the session: "I'm an athlete. That therapist has no idea what to do with me!"

Rather than go on being treated by someone in whom she had no confidence, Kristen on her own found a former semi-professional athlete whose physical therapy practice centered on athletes. Kristen went back to her doctor, saying, "She knows what I want to achieve. Please endorse her so I can get my insurance to pay for the sessions." The doctor concurred without argument, and immediately after her surgery, Kristen began working productively with the more aggressive therapist.

treatment. Most patients do better with ongoing support and attention. You'll also want to be sure you're working with a dietitian who is accepted and covered by your health insurance policy.

### Look for PTs or OTs who are suited to your background, attitude, and philosophy of recovery.

Physical and occupational therapy programs are by no means alike. A therapist's practice may be based on any of a wide variety of theories and employ a distinctive (and in some cases controversial) technique, or use a combination of several different techniques. Your doctor will play a major role in choosing the type of therapy best suited to your case, but you should certainly ask your doctor to take into account your own beliefs, experience, background, and attitude toward recovery. The story in the box on page 232 is a good case in point.

### Keep in mind, in most cases it's not mandatory for a hospital patient to participate in recreational therapy activities.

If you're feeling trapped, isolated, and miserable during your hospital stay, dancing and drawing pictures may not be what you think you need. Maybe you'd rather just talk your problems over with someone directly. If so, politely decline the recreational therapist's invitations, and ask your own physician for a referral to a psychologist, psychiatrist, or other mental health professional.

### If you're working with a speech-language pathologist or an audiologist in the hospital, ask about involving the people closest to you in your exercises.

Soon you'll be home and will need all the help you can get to communicate with your family and others in your household. By participating in your oral or auditory rehabilitation exercises, the people around you can come to understand more about your difficulties in communication and see what you are doing to overcome your problems. They learn the skills and pick up the clues they need to help you make yourself understood and ease the transition to a normal life.

**Before scheduling any test involving the use of radiation or radioactive materials, ask questions about shielding and other safety measures to protect patients.**
You may be handed, mailed, or faxed a pamphlet about the safety of the equipment and/or dyes used, with reassuring data about the lack of long-term adverse effects on patients who have had the procedure. If you haven't undergone any sort of test using radiation in many years, you may not be aware that the machines in use today work very effectively using far less radiation that was necessary in the past. I think you will find the staff at the radiology center both knowledgeable and willing to address any safety issues that you raise.

**Before the X-ray starts, check to be sure that protective lead shielding is in place.**
This is the job of the X-ray technician, of course, but there's no reason why the patient shouldn't also watch out to be sure this essential step isn't skipped. If the X-ray technician is going to take a picture of your arm, for example, you need to be covered with a lead-lined apron from the thyroid at the base of your neck down to your groin. If you are in a hospital room or recovery room and the person in bed next to you is set to be X-rayed with a portable machine, make sure the technician or a nurse has set up a lead screen between you and the other patient.

**Tell the MRI technician if you have any claustrophobic tendencies.**
This is a common problem for MRI patients. An experienced professional technician will be able to take measures to reduce your anxiety level and increase your comfort before you go into the MRI. You do need to make the technician aware of your panic potential ahead of time, however. If you think you have any tendency at all to "freak out" during the exam, be up-front about it. You don't want your MRI to be ruined and need to be repeated because you underestimated your innate claustrophobia and were unable to remain still for the necessary length of time.

**Before any sort of test that may be uncomfortable or noisy, ask about the possibility of bringing in headphones to listen to music or a book on tape.**

In the boxed list of questions on page 231 I suggest asking your MRI technician about using headphones during the test, both to distract you and to block out the loud banging, clicking, and whirring sounds coming from the machine. You may want to ask the same question of your cardiovascular technologist before your angiogram (it's not a noisy test, but it can certainly be unpleasant) or of the assistants who prepare you for oral surgery, especially if it involves drilling.

**Always assume that you'll have to wait a while before a test begins, so bring a book or some other quiet amusement to help pass the time.**

Otherwise, you'll doubtless sit there growing more anxious by the minute.

**If you've come into the hospital through the emergency room or have been hospitalized for any problem that affects your ability to get around on your own, ask if testing equipment can be brought to your hospital bed.**

Usually technicians like to administer tests in their specialized testing rooms and so prefer to transport you in a wheelchair or on a gurney. However, many hospitals also have portable X-ray machines or other diagnostic equipment that can be brought to the patient's room. It's worth asking about, especially if you're in pain and want to limit the amount of times you are picked up and moved from place to place.

**If in preparation for a colonoscopy or any of a variety of other gastroinstestinal procedures, you are directed to drink a large quantity of a fluid called GoLytely or NuLytely, ask if it can be flavored.**

GoLytely (or NuLytely) causes your digestive tract to empty itself of all food you've eaten recently. It's typically given before any test or procedure that involves the introduction of instruments or other foreign elements into your gastrointestinal tract. Unflavored, these drinks taste simply foul—sewage water seems like a nice soft drink by comparison. But they're also available with a flavoring (cherry, lemon-lime, or pineapple) to make the stuff go down a little easier. If not offered the flavored type, take it from me, this is definitely something worth asking about!

## When technicians use terms unfamiliar to you, politely interrupt to ask what they're talking about.

It's stressful enough to be alone in a room full of strange and menacing looking machinery, but it's even worse when you hear the white-coat-wearing stranger behind the lead shield talking about you to some other stranger using words you don't understand. Debby's experience, described in the box below, is an example of the sort of thing no patient should have to put up with from hospital technicians.

*After eleven months* of unsuccessful fertility treatments Debby was ecstatic to learn that her pregnancy test had finally come back positive. Her doctor told her to schedule a uterine ultrasound as soon as possible, to confirm that the embryo had implanted and was developing normally. Debby diligently followed all the pre-test instructions, arriving at the diagnostic center at the right time, with a full bladder, and filling out all the paperwork. She disrobed from the waist down and was covered with a paper sheet, and then waited patiently on the examining table.

Without a word of greeting, the technologist came in, covered her abdomen with a blue gel and began passing the transducer over her to conduct the exam. A fuzzy image soon appeared on the computer screen next to the examining table. Debby was full of questions: "Is that my baby? Do things look normal? What are those measurements you're making?"

Instead of answering her, the technician turned to another staff member and remarked, "No fetal pole." He noted some measurements on the computer and then walked out. He'd never even looked directly at her. Debby knew something was seriously wrong, but why wouldn't anyone tell her what it was? "What did those words mean—'No fetal pole,'" Debby wondered. On her way out, she asked the receptionist, who told her with a shrug, "You'll have to ask your doctor."

It was several hours before Debby's doctor called back with the news she suspected and had been dreading. Her pregnancy had not implanted successfully. The words "no fetal pole" meant that the technician had not seen traces of a spinal chord, the first part of the fetus to develop in pregnancy.

"Of course it was disappointing to find out that I wasn't pregnant," Debby said, "but it was made even harder by the way the technician talked about it in front of me without bothering to explain to me what he was seeing."

Debby eventually did get pregnant and have a healthy baby—but she never used that diagnostic center for any of the tests she needed during that pregnancy or afterward.

### If you can't figure out what a particular technologist does by his or her title, ask for clarification.

Let's say you're sent to a room in the hospital for tests, and the person you encounter there introduces himself to you as an interventional venapuncturist. Would you think you were meeting: A doctor who perforates blood vessels? The technician who draws your blood? A representative of the Red Cross blood drive? Count Dracula?

Okay, I admit it, this abstruse title is actually a product of my imagination—and I hope it will remain so. If you do come across it, however, the term would probably refer to the technician who draws your blood. You get a boost in your ability to guess what medical terms mean if you've ever studied Latin or Greek, the two most common sources of root meanings in medicine. But you shouldn't need applied linguistics to know who will be doing what to you in the hospital. All you should have to do is ask. (Actually, you should never *have* to ask; they should be taught to introduce themselves first thing.)

Just say, "Excuse me, but could you please tell me who you are and what it is you're about to do?"

If the answer comes back, "Ask your doctor," then you say, "Yes, I really think I need to do that before I have this procedure." That will put a halt to the proceedings and give you the opportunity to find out if the test is truly necessary or beneficial in your case.

**If you must go again and again to same diagnostic center, ask for the technicians you've found to be gentle and effective.**
Use your familiarity with the center and its staff to your advantage. The trick is to keep track of names and faces, and observe closely who is best at doing what. Then ask that person directly, "What's the best way to schedule my next procedure so that I'm sure to get you again?" Like everyone else, medical staff members like to be recognized and appreciated for their work. In most cases a technician will be more than willing to help you connect with him or her again. The stories in the box on page 239 demonstrate how other patients have done this.

**Try to get consistency at all stages of the health care experience.**
Whenever you have to go to the hospital, not only do you want the same technicians that you know and like, but you also want the same doctors, nurses, and surgical support staff, if you can get them. Consistency can definitely affect the quality of care, not just your comfort level. When an anesthesiologist knows you already, it's not just your name and history that he or she will find it easier to keep in mind, but a whole range of experience that comes from having watched you, for example, react under anesthesia or improve when prescribed certain drugs but not others. When your caregivers have seen you before and know they'll be seeing you again, they think of you as more than just another patient, someone to be worked on and forgotten about the next day. They'll greet you and ask about what's going on in your life, and let you know they'll be looking out for this or that special problem they know you have. That can make the difference between just a so-so hospital experience and one that really speeds you along the road to recovery.

***During her time*** in fertility treatment, Amy was required to report to the hospital's blood drawing lab each morning for ten to twelve days out of each menstrual cycle, to have a blood sample taken and analyzed for hormonal levels. After a few months she came to know all the phlebotomists who worked there, and she learned who could always got a good stick on the first try, who had a gentle touch, who would wait for her to get comfortable and remember to ask her which arm she preferred. Though the daily blood drawing was never a pleasant experience, it certainly became less stressful when performed by a technician she liked and trusted.

**********

***I have a patient*** with liver disease who often comes to the hospital where I work for an upper endoscopy (viewing his esophagus and stomach with a fiber-optic scope). He's known as a "difficult IV stick"—that is, getting the IV line started on him is a challenge. He wants only a certain doctor to do his IV because he likes that doctor's touch. Now he's got us so well trained to respond to his preferences that the minute we see his name on the schedule, we make sure that his preferred doctor will be on.

## Know what to expect when you are sent to a specialized area of the hospital.

The two particular specialized units I'll discuss here are the intensive care unit (ICU) and the cardiac care unit (CCU). Your hospital may also have a specialized unit for cancer patients or a specialized unit for patients who need some other form of advanced care, but I have picked these two units as examples because they can be found in most large hospitals.

*Intensive care unit (ICU).* "Intensive care" has a scary sound to it. When do you go to the ICU? When you need close monitoring of your blood pressure, pulse, blood oxygen levels, and consciousness. In the ICU, the monitoring goes on from minute to minute rather than hour to hour or four times a day. Depending on the hospital, you may even have a specialized doctor called an *intensivist* overseeing your care in the ICU. That doctor might be an anesthesiologist, a surgeon, a cardiologist, a pulmonary specialist—intensivists come from a number of medical disciplines—but he or she will also be highly trained in critical care and may even be board certified in that area.

Staff members who work in the ICU are good at staying calm during events that make other people frantic. Upon awaking to find themselves in the ICU, some patients become hysterical, even though their long-term prognosis may be good. More commonly, though, patients in the ICU are not clear-headed enough to understand where they are and how badly they're injured or how ill they are. In either case, ICU staff members are trained to respond in ways that both comfort and take care of the patient's immediate medical needs.

*Cardiac care unit (CCU).* The CCU is like an ICU for the heart. The issues are the same here as for the ICU, but all patients in the CCU have heart-related problems.

You will probably find that the atmosphere in the CCU is more relaxed than in the ICU; the staff deliberately try to keep things low-key because many people there have just had heart attacks or come out of open-heart surgery. They want their patients to be comfortable and, at least initially, they try to keep patients' mental, physical, and emotional stimulation down to a minimum. The CCU staff got very annoyed with a friend of mine who came to visit her stockbroker boyfriend, a heart attack victim at the age of thirty-six, bringing copies of *The Wall Street Journal* and *Investor's Business Daily* each time she came.

# CHAPTER 11

# Leaving the Hospital ... and Beyond

A t last! It's time to go home, back to your own cozy bed, and not too long afterward (so you hope), back to your normal routine. But first, a few (okay, more than a few) tips and suggestions to make sure that everything gets on the right track after your discharge from the hospital.

### Get out of the hospital as quickly as you can stand to go.

This is an important safety tip, because the hospital is truly "the Land of Germs." If your doctor is wise, he or she will do everything to speed you out the front door the instant you no longer need hospital care. You might think it's a bad thing not to have the services of nurses, bringing your meals and helping you bathe, but just remember, you're also depriving all those hospital germs of the opportunity to bring you some interesting new infections. Once you consider the prevalence of hospital-borne infections, you'll realize that the inconveniences of being at home are far outweighed by the safety factor.

### Get your discharge instructions in writing.

Most hospitals will provide you with a written sheet—and quite possibly, multiple sheets of densely worded, single-spaced type—with the instructions you are supposed follow the first few days or weeks at home. These may include

- How to bathe.
- When and how to change your dressings.

- What medications to take and when to take them.
- Any exercises, stretches, or therapeutic activities to practice.
- Any activity to avoid, and for how long.
- How to recognize signs of infection or other complications.
- When to call your doctor.
- Date, time, and place of your next appointment.

Read through everything carefully before you leave the hospital. (You may be required to sign the form and leave a copy with the hospital.) If there's anything you don't understand or feel you cannot do on your own, raise the issue with your doctor. Don't go home in a state of confusion about *anything,* because when it's three in the morning (and it's *always* three in the morning when anything goes wrong, isn't it?), you won't want to find yourself unable to get a quick yes or no to the question, "Is it normal for me to … [have whatever symptoms I'm having]?"

**Be sure you understand your medication schedule before you leave the hospital.**
The medications you take at home may not be same as those given in hospital, or the pills may be the same, but the schedule may be different. In any case, you need to be clear on your instructions. Find out, for example, if "four times a day" means exactly every six hours over a twenty-four-hour period, in which case you will need to wake up at least once in the middle of an eight-hour night's sleep to stick with the program, or if it's perfectly okay to take the first pill when you wake up, the next one around lunchtime, the third one in the late afternoon, and the last one of the day just before you go to bed.

**If you're put on a medication schedule that will be difficult to follow, find out whether it can be changed.**
Sometimes a doctor doesn't take into account how hard it is for you to wake up three times a night to take your medication. Occasionally, the instructions for taking one medication will pose a conflict with those for another: For example, you are put on two medications, each

to be taken around the same times of the day, but one is supposed to be taken with a meal, while the other is supposed to be taken on an empty stomach, and your stomach must remain empty for at least an hour afterward. It's frequently the case that a doctor can modify the schedule or substitute a similar drug that's more practical to take, with no loss of medical effectiveness. In any case, there's no downside in asking.

**Discuss any new medications you'll be taking—especially narcotics—with the prescribing doctor before your discharge, and again, with the pharmacist who dispenses it.** Find out if there are any extra tips about taking the medication that you should be aware of: for example, "To minimize the possibility of stomach distress, avoid citrus fruits and juices while on this medication," or "Do not drive while on this medication." These sorts of advisories may be found on the patient package insert that by federal law must accompany all drugs, but many patients (especially those of us who are starting to have trouble making out that tiny type!) find these jargon-filled sheets hard to understand. One of the specific questions you want to ask of both the prescribing doctor and your pharmacist is how the new drug will interact with any of the other drugs you are taking. Then you'll know which side effects to be most vigilant about reporting.

**If you're on multiple medications, make a weekly calendar for your home use, showing the name of what you're taking, the dose, the time of day to take each dose, and other notes.** You might want to set it up with columns for the days and rows for each of the medication-taking time slots, with a check-off box next to each dose, as shown in the example on page 244. If someone at home can design your calendar on the computer for you, based on your medication instructions, you can show it to your doctor to be reviewed for accuracy even before you are discharged.

**When you fill your prescriptions for the medications you will use at home, before you leave the pharmacy, compare**

**the drug names, dosages, and schedules to the information
on your list.**

If you find any discrepancies—for example, it looks to you as though
you will be taking less of the painkiller than you thought you were
going to get—ask the pharmacist to double-check and, if necessary,
call your doctor to confirm that you're getting what was ordered.

Most patients just released from the hospital will send a friend or
family member to the pharmacy to fill their prescriptions, or they will
have the pharmacy deliver. In either case, it's important for the person handling the transaction to check to be sure you're getting just

| Sample Medication Calendar for the First Week Home from the Hospital | | | |
|---|---|---|---|
| Time / Day | 7 a.m. | 8 a.m. | 7 p.m. |
| Sunday | ❑ 500 mg Augmentin | ❑ 6 tablets, 5 mg ea. Prednisone, take with food or milk | ❑ 500 mg Augmentin |
| Monday | ❑ 500 mg Augmentin | ❑ 5 tablets, 5 mg ea. Prednisone, take with food or milk | ❑ 500 mg Augmentin |
| Tuesday | ❑ 500 mg Augmentin | ❑ 4 tablets, 5 mg ea. Prednisone, take with food or milk | ❑ 500 mg Augmentin |
| Wednesday | ❑ 500 mg Augmentin | ❑ 3 tablets, 5 mg ea. Prednisone, take with food or milk | ❑ 500 mg Augmentin |
| Thursday | ❑ 500 mg Augmentin | ❑ 2 tablets, 5 mg ea. Prednisone, take with food or milk | ❑ 500 mg Augmentin |
| Friday | ❑ 500 mg Augmentin | ❑ 1 tablet, 5 mg Prednisone, take with food or milk | ❑ 500 mg Augmentin |
| Saturday | ❑ 500 mg Augmentin | | ❑ 500 mg Augmentin |

what the doctor ordered. It's very annoying—not to mention wasteful of valuable time—to have to go back to exchange the wrong drug for the right one.

**If your post-discharge medication regimen is complicated, use organizer boxes, electronic devices, or reminder services to keep you on top of things.**
Medical supply companies, like Royal Medical Supply (on the web at *www.a-royalmed.com* or call 877-22-ROYAL), sell a variety of pill organizer boxes. One has movable, color-coded dividers that allow you to group your doses by date and time; another has only two compartments but also has a built-in electronic alarm clock that you can set to sound at the appropriate times; a third is a combination wristwatch and pill holder that can store up to thirty small pills as well keep time and beep at your preset intervals.

You may not have to buy anything if you already own a Palm Pilot or any other PDA (personal digital assistant). Most of these are designed to download calendar entries from your home computer and beep for anything you want to be reminded about. You can also buy a pill reminder program specifically designed for your Palm Pilot or for any other major brand of PDA.

If you don't own a Palm Pilot but you are a computer user, then check out the free web-based service offered through Mr. Wake-Up at *www.mrwakeup.com*. Click on the tab labeled "Dr. Dose." You will be shown a calendar that you can click on to set the dates and times for which you want reminders set, and a box to type in the name of the medication. You provide a telephone number for notification, and the service will then automatically call you and play a message telling you to take your erythromycin or whatever drug you specified. You can also set Dr. Dose to send a text message to your computer, beeper, or text-receiving cell phone.

**Don't add any herbal products to your medication schedule without your doctor's approval.**
In Chapter 3, I discussed why you must inform your doctor about any herbal products you're taking before surgery. It's every bit as

necessary—maybe even more important—to do so when you're taking drugs designed to help you recover from surgery at home. As discussed on pages 53-55, a number of different herbals have an anticoagulant effect, that is, they promote bleeding—not at all desirable for most post-surgical patients. The herb dong quai has been shown to counteract the effects of tamoxifen, which many women must take after breast cancer treatment. Never accept the reassurances of an herbalist, naturopath, or other alternative therapist who lacks a degree in pharmacology or medicine; find out what a qualified medical expert has to say before tampering in any way with your medication regimen.

**Diligently follow your post-discharge instructions about changing your bandage and checking your wound for infection.**
If you have any suspicion that your wound looks infected—redness, swelling, increasing pain, oozing pus—call your doctor immediately.

**If you'll need in-home care, know your options.**
Before your discharge you will probably be visited by a social services worker from the hospital staff who will go over your options if you need in-home care. (If the hospital doesn't send someone to help you make these arrangements, ask your doctor to refer you to a social services agency that will advise you.)

This social worker may put you in touch with your local office of the Visiting Nurse Association, a not-for-profit organization that helps patients find qualified in-home nursing care (RNs, LPNs, LVNs or APNs, as needed) or you may be referred to a private, for-profit agency that can supply you with a home health aide (what hospitals call UAP for "unlicensed assistive personnel," who may or may not have any specialized training in nursing tasks).

Depending on the level of care needed, you may want to have your nurse (or nurses) or your home health aide(s) live in or live out; you may opt for round-the-clock shifts, occasional check-in visits, or anything in between.

You may not need any specialized skills at all, just someone who can cook for you and bring you your meals and help you in and out of bed for a week or two, until you're back on your feet. In that case, perhaps a family member, a good friend, or a combination of friends and relatives could work out a schedule to be available to help out in the first few days that you're home.

After you've drawn up a plan for the sort of home health care provider you will hire, ask your doctor to review it to make sure it's adequate to the level of medical care needed. This step will also help you when it comes to insurance coverage, discussed below.

## Find out whether your insurance will cover your in-home care, and if necessary, look into subsidized services.

Unless you have already added a long-term nursing care rider to your health care plan (and very few subscribers think to do so), you will probably discover that your insurance will not pay for the in-home nurses you need. You can argue and argue that otherwise you would have to stay longer in the hospital at a cost to your insurance company of many hundreds of dollars a day, and that it's in their interest to pay for your home care, but in the end you will be told, "rules are rules."

In some cases a standard health insurance policy will pay for in-home care for a limited period of time, under certain medical circumstances (home IV medication for AIDS or cancer patients, for example). You will normally need your doctor to write a letter to the insurance company certifying that you meet its medical criteria for in-home care. However, in some cases you may qualify for state subsidized care. Some states allow home nursing for a limited time for elderly or low-income patients.

If you were in a teaching hospital, find out whether the hospital runs a program in which medical students provide free or low-cost in-home services. Especially in inner-city areas, some medical schools have set up social service programs to give students some practical educational experience and a chance to serve the surrounding community at the same time. Students will either donate their services or be paid a nominal wage; patients (who are usually referred to as "clients" once they are at home) will pay nothing or pay on a sliding scale based on their means.

There are also charitable organizations that serve patients' home care needs. If you are elderly, find out whether your city or town has any sort of senior center that sends out volunteers to make regular visits to the homebound in the area. A Meals-on-Wheels plan might be all that you need to help you out until you are able to cook for yourself again. Your hospital social worker should know what sort of services are available to you.

If you don't qualify for any free or subsidized program, but are still too strapped for funds to pay for needed in-home care out of pocket, then don't be shy about asking friends, relatives, and neighbors for the short-term help you need. You will undoubtedly be gratified to discover how much people are willing to do for each other when called upon—and make clear, when you bring up your need, that one day you hope to be able to do a good deed for them in return.

**Consider what clothing would be most comfortable during your recovery at home.**
You don't want to wear anything that is tight around the site of your incision or pulls at your dressings. This simple, commonsense advice is all too often neglected in the larger scheme of things. Patients assume they'll wear the same clothes they came in to go home from the hospital, only to discover as they try to pull on that tight pair of jeans that it hurts too much to even try to zip up the fly. If you've had abdominal surgery, you're going to want to wear something loose around your waist (for women, a shift dress; for men, a big, baggy pair of overalls). Women who have had heart surgery shouldn't plan on wearing a bra for a while to come, and when they do go back to wearing one, it should be one made of a soft, stretchy fabric without any underwiring or rigid construction. Both women and men will want to sleep in a nightshirt rather than pajamas with an elastic waistband. If you don't have these items of clothing at home, then send a friend to the store to pick something up for you, or put in a catalog order over the phone, and if your discharge date is looming, ask for next-day air delivery.

**Find out how long you should wait before driving.**
This bit of information may be buried somewhere in your multi-page discharge instructions. Or you may find written in big, bold type:

"Don't drive for six weeks" and think to yourself, "That's nuts! I'm perfectly fine to drive." But it's never good idea to jump back behind the wheel after surgery without checking with your doctor first. You may be told that the six-week prohibition is just a precaution, and that it can be reduced to three weeks in your particular case. Or you may learn that six weeks is the absolute minimum you must wait, and that to avoid danger of fainting or dizziness, you will need to pass certain neurological tests before you can drive again. If you're restricted from driving, make sure you understand the safety reasoning behind the ban; that way you won't not be tempted to violate it and end up causing an accident that could put you, and perhaps innocent others, in far worse shape than you were in before your surgery.

### Make arrangements to get whatever home medical equipment you need during your recovery.

Medical supply companies can rent or sell you practically anything you need: wheelchairs, canes, walkers, handrails for home installation, shower seats, hydrotherapy attachments for your bathtub, adjustable beds (like the one you had in the hospital), triangular bed wedges to keep your head or some other body part elevated, disposable bed protectors so that your oozing wound won't ruin your nice sheets, and hundreds more items. If you have access to the Internet, all you need to do is go to any comprehensive search engine, type in the name of the device or mobility aid you need, hit "enter" and wait for the thousands of "hits" to pop up on your screen. If you don't have an Internet browser, then try the Yellow Pages under the heading "medical equipment."

For patients who are not supposed to lift their arms above their heads (an instruction commonly given to those recovering from heart surgery), I recommend getting a long-handled grabbing stick. This is a gadget with a pincer claw-like device on the end of a handle. With it you can get items down from shelves above you without reaching up, and you can also bring things over to you without getting out of bed. Most medical supply stores carry them; I found a good online source at Senior Shops at *http://www.seniorshops.com/reachers1.html*.

A bedside tray of adjustable height on wheels is another great item for any patient just home from the hospital. The Signals catalog (*www.GiftCatalog.com* or call 800-669-9696) has a nice one that is not a bad piece of furniture, even when you're not sick (Rolling Reader's Table, item #78958).

**If you wish to incorporate some form of alternative physical therapy into your at-home recovery plan, discuss the matter thoroughly with your doctor.**

Describe to your doctor in detail what you'd like to do. If it's a yoga exercise, you might want your yoga teacher to supply you with drawings or even a video showing the movement you will be making. That way your doctor can be sure your program does not violate any temporary or permanent restrictions on your movements after surgery. If you will be seeing a chiropractor, massage therapist, acupuncturist, or other therapist who will be manipulating your body, you might ask that person to consult directly with your doctor and then have your doctor advise you about any safety concerns. What you *don't* want is to have to rely on the alternative therapist's own assessment of the health risks for a person in your condition; unless that therapist is also a qualified expert in that field of medicine, he or she is not in a position to provide reliable information.

**Consider whether your doctor may be biased toward a brand-name drug or source of post-surgical therapy services.**

Believe it or not (I have a feeling you do), pharmaceutical companies can influence doctors. While you're in the hospital, you might receive medication you are told you must continue taking after your discharge. Let's say you get a prescription for a specific brand from your doctor. Ask if that's precisely the medication you have been getting, or if it was it another brand, or perhaps a generic version. If you were given a generic drug in the hospital, ask why your doctor recommends the change. There may or may not be a medical reason.

Whenever you get a prescription for a brand name, ask your doctor if you can use the generic version instead. If the answer is no, pose the same question to the pharmacist when you go to fill the prescription. You might get a different answer, which may simply mean that the pharmacist has more current knowledge of the available generics than the doctor does. Then again, the doctor might have a non-medical reason for recommending the brand.

Doctors can also have financial interests in laboratories, physical therapy clinics, and other medical businesses, in which case they might want to steer you in that direction. Ask if you really need to use that particular product or service. What doctors are ethically required to do in these case is to disclose any corporate relationship that may bias them in one direction and then offer you alternatives. If you believe the doctor isn't following these rules, you may want to follow up by phoning the lab or clinic and asking to speak to someone in a management position. Ask, "Does Dr. [Whoever] have a business relationship with your facility?" If the answer is yes, you can conclude that the doctor is more interested in his own financial gain than in his obligations to you as a patient.

**In the event that your hospital stay has turned into a horror story, you and/or your patient advocate will need to follow up your complaints with actions—including legal action, if necessary.**

In Chapter 5, I discussed the need to keep a log and all supporting documentation as evidence of any malpractice you may have been subjected to while in the hospital. It's not often possible to pursue your case while you are laid up; action must usually wait until you're feeling well enough to stand up for your rights.

Once you are at home, you may gain the time and perspective you need to evaluate your hospital experience, identify the culpable party or parties, and determine what remedies are open to you. There are medical investigative bodies and physicians disciplinary boards, both within the hospital and in the larger community; there is also the national Joint Commission on Accreditation of Healthcare Organizations (JCAHO). (See the next tip for more information about filing a complaint.) In some cases, criminal charges may be warranted (for example, if it can be proven that the surgeon was operating under a suspended medical license or if he lied to you about his qualifications); and of course, there are lawyers who will file a malpractice suit on your behalf.

Be aware that you must act within a set period of time, the statute of limitations, after the incident to initiate legal proceedings against a defendant. Find out what the statute is in your case. Usually you have a minimum of a year, and in many cases, several years. Although you don't want to let time slip away and lose the opportunity to interview witnesses and collect documentation, you don't want to rush to the courts, either. Give yourself time to think matters through and carefully weigh your options before going ahead with a case.

*A woman in the hospital* for a hysteroscopy faced grave complications. Her gynecologist was using a relatively new piece of equipment that fills the uterus with a solution to clean out fibroid tumors. During the procedure, the meter that measures fluid input and outtake malfunctioned. It is absolutely essential that body fluids be kept at an equilibrium during a process of this nature: If the doctor pumps three liters into the patient, three liters must be flushed out. Operating room personnel are like commercial pilots: They rely heavily on the accuracy of their gauges to avoid obstacles in their path. The surgical staff may have looked at the malfunctioning meter, but what they failed to do was to monitor the patient's own reaction to the steady buildup of fluids within her uterus. First, her skin began to turn blue, and then she puffed up like a balloon. She was headed for congestive heart failure—and worse. By the time someone noticed her condition, she was so swollen that the anesthesiologist couldn't even intubate her. Some among the OR staff broke down, certain that they would lose her. The anesthesiologist started to cry. Another anesthesiologist working nearby heard the commotion down the hall and ran in to see if he could help. When he saw the patient's low blood oxygen levels, he realized there was no time to waste: If she didn't get a breathing tube down her within the next minute or two, she would die. He grabbed the first general surgeon he saw, who, fortunately, was able to make a breathing hole in her throat before brain death set in. After pumping oxygen into her as quickly as possible, they transferred her to intensive care—but she didn't show any signs of waking up.

> For hours the ICU nurses kept close tabs on her. First, the flicker of an eye, then a squeeze of a hand, and then, at last, consciousness. Her return to a completely normal state was nearly miraculous—the end of a medical trauma, but the beginning of a legal one.

## File your complaint against the hospital with the Joint Committee on Accreditation of Healthcare Organizations.

In Chapter 2, I explained how the JCAHO undertakes periodic reviews of every accredited hospital in America. It also runs a system that takes complaints about the facilities it has accredited. You can send your complaint by email to complaint@jcaho.org, by telephone to the complaint hotline at 800-994-6610, by fax to the attention of the Office of Quality Monitoring at 630-792-5636, or by regular mail addressed to the Office of Quality Monitoring, JCAHO, One Renaissance Boulevard, Oakbrook Terrace, IL 60181. Summarize your complaint in one to two pages and include the full name, street address, city, and state of the hospital or health care organization in question.

## Examine your hospital bills for errors and question any charges for drugs and services you did not receive.

A recent study has shown that up to 20 percent of hospital bills are fraught with error, either overcharging or charging for services never performed. Sometimes you will find that you receive a bill for a piece of surgical equipment that was never used, but the charge is still considered legitimate. Why? It was "on hand" in case the doctor needed it. The same goes for fees associated with a doctor who was present for a surgery, but did not perform any of the operation.

Myvesta.org is a nonprofit, Internet-based financial counseling and services organization that offers a series of tips for spotting errors on your bill and keeping costs contained. Among them are:

- When in the hospital, keep track of tests, services and medications. Compare them to the final itemized bill to see if you're being overcharged.

- Anytime your doctor writes a prescription, ask for free samples of the medication.
- Always find out if you have the option of taking a lower-cost generic substitute.

Myvesta.org goes into a lot more detail in its free publication, *Coping With Medical Bills*. You can download it from the website at ***www.Myvesta.org***.

### Be prepared to appeal to your insurance company when you are denied coverage.

If you feel you've been cheated out of coverage you believe your policy was supposed to provide, you'll be better positioned to fight for reimbursement at the successful conclusion of your treatment. You should be able to produce letters from your doctors, studies, or other documents supporting your contention that there was no safe course other than to perform that procedure at the time it was done. You generally don't pay your surgeon's bills in advance, so you should find him or her highly motivated to help you pursue your appeal with your insurance company.

If your insurance company has turned you down on the basis of the "experimental" nature of your procedure, it's important to show how widespread the treatment has become. Your surgeon should certainly be able to assist you in gathering such data.

Always make copies of everything you send to your insurance company.

### If your hospital bill goes to a collection agency, know your legal rights.

Don't be intimidated: There are both federal and state laws to protect you. For a good, plain-English summary of the protections in the law, visit the website of the 'Lectric Law Library at ***www.lectlaw.com/ files/cos26.htm***. You can't be harassed at home or threatened with exposure in public, nor can a debt collector contact you at work.

If you are subject to any debt collection action in violation of the law, you might want to go to ***www.gottrouble.com/legal/ consumer_law/debt_collection.html*** to find out what to do next. You can get a referral to a consumer rights attorney in your local area or pose a question to be answered through the medium of cyberspace.

## If your hospital experience was a good one, then give compliments where they are due.

You probably got this book because you're concerned about protecting yourself from things that can go wrong in the hospital. I sincerely hope nothing did. If, instead of having to keep a sharp eye out to prevent yourself from falling victim to medical mishaps, you found your care to be consistently attentive and warm-spirited, you should certainly express your compliments to the staff. A thank you note is always a nice gesture. You may send the letter to all the nurses at the nursing station on your floor, or address it to any particular nurse who has earned your praise. A copy to the hospital administrator's office would be a nice idea, too.

Looking after hospital patients is a tough job, and those of us who do it really do need all the encouragement we can get!

# Sample Medical Emergency ID Card

Every person should keep a wallet card with essential emergency contact information, along the lines of the sample below.

---

**Sample Medical Emergency Card**

EMERGENCY INFORMATION FOR
Mary Elizabeth Somebody
0000 Somewhere Street, Apt. E-Z
Anytown, ST  00000
H – 202-555-4321; O – 202-555-9090
DOB: 12/19/73   Medical note: Contact lens wearer
Emergency contact (husband): John Bigshot
O – 202-555-8888; cell – 817-555-9876
For medical history contact Dr. Maxwell S. Hammer
O – 202-555-6789; after-hrs. – 202-555-0505

---

If you have any chronic condition such as asthma, diabetes, or epilepsy, or a severe drug allergy, you might want to note it on the card; however, the safer course of action is to wear a medical alert bracelet or pendant identifying the condition and providing the number of a 24-hour monitoring center that keeps a copy of any medical instructions you want given out in an emergency. (See Chapter 9, page 184 for information about ordering medical alert tags from the Medic Alert Foundation.)

Laminate your card with plastic sheets, which you can buy in any office supply store. Check it periodically to see if anything needs updating, especially the name and phone number of the doctor you want contacted first.

In Chapter 9 you will also find information about creating other cards and documents of value in an emergency: a current medications card to carry with you and a patient medical history to keep readily accessible (perhaps in a drawer by your telephone).

# Common Outpatient (Same Day) Procedures

Generally, it's to your advantage—medically and financially—to get in and out of the hospital as quickly as possible. Surgeries done with a laparoscopic incision using a fiber-optic scope are far less invasive than the "open" version that required at least an overnight stay in the hospital. Lasers and other tools now used in many surgeries and tests have made them much simpler, safer procedures as well.

On the other hand, some procedures that sound simple may require admission because of the type of complications that could develop. For example, a doctor may sometimes keep a patient overnight to watch for unusual swelling after casting an arm or leg.

This appendix describes includes the most commonly performed procedures that, under normal circumstances, will not require an overnight stay in a hospital or clinic.

**ACL repair.** Surgery to repair or replace the anterior cruciate ligament in the knee, usually taking from two to five hours. The choice of anesthetic includes general, spinal, or epidural. The main problem with spinal or epidural anesthesia is that the surgery has the potential to be lengthy, so if you're a fidgety person or don't want to be concerned about being uncomfortable on the operating room table, opt for the general. The caveat is that you must be a good candidate for general anesthesia. Some patients ending up needing an overnight stay in the hospital as a result of the common side effects of the anesthesia. If it turns out that you're unable to take any food or liquid by mouth because of persistent vomiting or inability to void (urinate), be prepared to spend the night.

**Adenoidectomy.** Although removal of the adenoids is most often done on children, adults occasionally need it, too. It's advisable when the adenoids block the area where the eustachian tube enters the inside of the throat from the ear and become a source of frequent infection and other difficulties. It may be done with or without a tonsillectomy, although it's so commonly done with one that the procedures might be referred to jointly as a "T and A." These days an adenoidectomy is most often done under general anesthesia, but in the past the tendency was to use a local. The most pronounced post-operative effect is a sore throat—usually treated with Popsicles and ice cream and by staying away from acidic foods or rough foods, such as lemonade, hard bread, or crackers.

**Anal fistula or fissure removal.** Whether the procedure involves a fistula (an abnormal tract, or tunnel, between the skin and underlying structures) or fissure (a crack), it's usually short and can be done under any of several different types of anesthesia: a general, a local with sedatives, a spinal, or an epidural. Expect to lie either on your stomach—the prone position—or in the lithotomy position, which is the open-legged, feet-in-stirrups position that a woman assumes during a gynecological exam. No doubt about it, the procedure is a "pain in the butt," so be sure to take measures that reduce the pain afterward, as much as possible. Follow your doctor's instructions on eating and drinking things that will soften your stool, and take the laxatives your doctor will certainly prescribe.

**Bartholin's cyst removal.** This is a female problem involving a small collection of fluid at one of the Bartholin's glands at the vaginal opening. You have the full range of options on anesthesia—general, sedation, spinal, or epidural—but general or sedation are preferable because the procedure is relatively short in duration.

**Bladder biopsy or tumor removal.** If you've had blood in your urine or noticed a change in your urinary habits, this may be the procedure for you. (If you are a smoker you should be aware that you are at much increased risk of developing a malignant bladder tumor.) A bladder biopsy or tumor removal can be a short procedure, but it can take a long time if the tumor mass is large. Done with a scope inserted into the penis or urethra, the procedure can be done under general, spinal, or epidural anesthesia, or with a combination of sedation plus a local anesthetic, specifically, lidocaine jelly injected in the urethra.

**Bladder dilation.** Necessary for patients afflicted with interstitial cystitis, the symptoms of which are frequent urination, lower abdominal or pelvic pain, and even blood in the urine. The procedure involves distention of the bladder with a scope, and it can be performed under general, spinal, or epidural anesthesia. It's short—only twenty or thirty minutes—but hard to tolerate under sedation because it is painful.

**Bladder tumor removal.** See "Bladder biopsy."

**Breast biopsy.** Although this may be done on either a man or woman with an abnormal mass in the breast, the most common patient is a woman who has had a mass detected during a breast exam. If the mass was discovered during mammography, you may come in for the biopsy with a wire already inserted in your breast. A radiologist will insert the wire into the area where the mass was pinpointed on the film; this is called "needle localization." The surgeon doing the biopsy cuts down to where the wire ends, that is, the wire is just a marker. If the mass is easy to feel, your physician may simply mark the area with a pen rather than insert a wire. Regardless of the preparatory technique, the tissue removed in the operating room is sent to the laboratory for analysis. The procedure is usually done using local anesthesia with sedation. When you come in for the procedure, make sure you come prepared to stay in the hospital. It is possible that your physician will want to operate further, based upon the lab findings. *Note:* This possibility is something to discuss thoroughly with your surgeon in advance of the date of the procedure.

**Bunion removal.** The act of taking part of the bone from the big toe is, in itself, not a terrible experience. It is done under heavy sedation with numbing medicine in the foot. The long and difficult part is the many weeks you will need to be able to place weight on the affected foot and the even longer time until you are able to walk normally and return to athletic activities.

**Carpal tunnel release.** The carpal ligament is a band of tissue on the inside of your wrist. Because of repetitive motion or disease, for example, the carpal tunnel may get tight to the point where this ligament compresses nerves that run through that tunnel. The surgeon has to cut that band of tissue, a procedure that can now be done arthroscopically. A tiny scope with a razor on the end snips the band of tissue to complete the procedure, which takes only a few minutes. Alternatively, some surgeons use a scalpel and do an open procedure with a small incision. Either way, it's done with local anesthesia, a local with sedation, or an arm-numbing medicine. Some surgeons prefer to use just a local anesthetic because the procedure is so short and the area involved is so small.

**Cataract removal.** Usually taking an hour or less, this procedure is most often done on older patients, who tend to have other medical problems. Those other problems must be stabilized before the cataract surgery. Before the removal, anesthesia can be delivered in either of two ways: through a numbing injection, which can be given under the eye or around the lower eyelid—a retrobulbar block—or by putting drops in your eyes. Once the numbing medicine is in, not only should you feel nothing in that area, but you also won't have vision in that eye so you don't have to be concerned about seeing anything scary. (A drape ensures that your other eye doesn't have to see anything scary either.) Without question, cataract removal is one of those procedures for which you want to find a surgeon who does it a lot. If a surgeon has a reputation for doing as many as eight or nine a day, that's a plus.

**Cholecystectomy (removal of the gall bladder).** These days this procedure is almost always done by using a scope, which is inserted through a very small incision, so instead of being "sliced and diced," a patient has the gall bladder sucked out through a tube. It is a very common procedure in the United States, especially among the population that can be described by most or all of the "five F" risk factors: fair (fair skinned), flatulent (gassy), fat, forty (or over), and fertile. As with any laporoscopic surgery, patients may complain afterwards of shoulder pain, because the residual air that's pumped into the abdominal cavity tends to result in what's known as a "referred pain" to the shoulder. Before the procedure, ask your physician to prescribe a painkiller in case you suffer from that common side effect.

**Closed repair, fractured bone.** A closed repair, or closed reduction, means that the doctor won't cut you through your skin to repair your fracture or dislocation, but will sedate you or give you general anesthesia while he or she manipulates your joint to set the bone. (See also "Open repair, fractured bone.")

**Cystoscopy of bladder.** See "Bladder biopsy."

**D&C (dilatation and curettage).** This procedure is done for both diagnostic purposes and, in the event of miscarriage, to remove the products of conception. Because the painful part of the procedure is the dilatation (also called "dilation," meaning "widening") of the opening to the cervix, women typically receive sedation plus a paracervical block, that is, an injection given at two locations around the cervix to numb it completely. Some doctors prefer to use general anesthesia, or will use it upon the patient's request.

**Ear tube placement.** This procedure is usually performed on young children who have chronic ear infections, but occasionally adults will need it for the same reason. Done under general anesthesia, this short procedure involves cutting a tiny hole in the eardrum and inserting a small tube, which will allow the product of the infection (we professionals call it "goo") to drain out and/or keep the passage open to prevent further infection. Once the child has outgrown the tendency toward ear infections or the adult patient has established a track record of being infection free, the surgeon will remove the tube; that's another brief surgery done under general anesthesia. *Word of warning:* Any time your doctor does a procedure on you that involves the ears or eyes, you are at increased risk for nausea for vomiting. To avoid this unpleasant side effect, ask about using ReliefBand, described in Chapter 4 "All About Anesthesia."

**Eye muscle defect correction.** A number of kids have strabismus, or "lazy eye," which requires tightening eye muscles. An interesting aside to this discussion is that there is a hypothesis that patients who require this surgery are at increased risk of malignant hyperthermia (see Appendix E, "Glossary of Hospital Terms" for definition) under anesthesia. The evidence, however, is far from conclusive. Correction of an eye muscle problem will typically involve general anesthesia. Here again, I offer the same warning that you will find above regarding ear surgery: Any time your doctor does a procedure on you that involves the ears or eyes, you can expect severe nausea. Again, I recommend using the ReliefBand, referenced above.

**Hammertoe correction.** See "Bunion removal."

**Hemorrhoidectomy.** See "Anal fistula or fissure removal."

**Hernia repair.** The repair of a hernia—any bulging of tissue through an opening where an opening doesn't belong—can be done in the traditional, open way, using a surgical knife, then sewing the tissues back together, or through a scope. In the latter approach, the surgeon uses a gas to inflate the lower part of the abdomen, fixes the problem by using the scope, and then rejoins the tissues with staples. The chief advantage of the scope is the shortened recovery time in most cases. Options for anesthesia include general, spinal, epidural, or local with sedation, unless the hernia is strangulated. If so, the surgeon has to pull the tissue through a tight opening, which requires complete muscle relaxation under general anesthesia.

**Hysteroscopy.** The surgeon puts a scope into the uterus and fills it with fluid to take a look at the structures inside. This procedure is often performed to detect and remove fibroids or a septum (tissue dividing the uterus into two compartments). It can be done with sedation or under spinal or epidural anesthesia. This is a procedure in which the surgical staff must keep a close eye on the level of fluid going in and out of the body. (For a chilling example of what can go wrong if the fluid intake is not monitored properly, see the story in the box on page 252.)

**Joint arthroscopy.** "Arthro" means "joint" and "scopy" means looking with a scope. It can be done on the knee, shoulder, elbow, wrist, and so on, and the reason to use a scope is to try to avoid cutting the patient open. Scope procedures are more conducive to swift recovery than their open counterparts. Using the scope as a guide, the surgeon will use tiny cutting or shaving devices, for example, to do repairs. For knees, the anesthesia is usually general, epidural, or spinal; for shoulders, surgeons generally go with a general, but some will try it with an upper-extremity nerve block. (I recommend the suprascapular nerve block for shoulder arthroscopy. Ask your surgeon or the anesthesia department if it's offered where you plan to have the surgery. If not, you may want to change your plans and go somewhere else.)

**Kidney stone crushing or removal.** Known also as lithotripsy, this procedure can be performed using a number of different types of machines. In one common method you will lie on a table and, through use of X-rays, the doctor will find the precise location of the stone and then focus a beam on it to break it up. It *is* painful. You should receive either sedation or general anesthesia. Although not quite as common, another method involves putting a patient in a tank of water and sending shock waves through the water to break up stones. It's more involved and is done only on patients who have a single, small stone; it's usually performed under general anesthesia.

**Laparoscopy.** This is a general term for using a scope in the abdomen. Diagnostic laparoscopy might involve making a series of small incisions around the abdomen to examine internal structures and find out whether surgery is indicated. The surgeon pumps carbon dioxide or another gas into the abdomen to inflate it and look inside to get a complete picture. Another type of laparoscopy is corrective, that is, it's used to treat your problem, by, for example, removing a cyst or mass. The most common anesthesia approach is general.

**Laryngoscopy.** This involves using a scope to examine the larynx, inserting it through the mouth, so the otolaryngologist (ear-nose-throat specialist, or ENT) can examine your vocal cords or the structures in your voice box and windpipe to see if you have any abnormalities. It usually requires general anesthesia. Now consider this: You obviously need a breathing tube (that is, you must be intubated) if you are under general anesthesia, but you also have a scope in your throat for the procedure, so the two small lines run side by side. The sort of work calls for a close team effort by your ENT and your anesthesiologist.

**LASIK.** The term is an abbreviation for laser-assisted in situ keratomileusis, a procedure that has become very popular for correcting both nearsightedness and farsightedness because the results are almost immediate. There is very little, if any, pain associated with the procedure, which is done after anesthetic drops are put in the eyes. The surgeon uses an instrument called a microkeratome to cut a thin flap in the cornea. After folding the flap back, he uses a laser to remove a little bit of corneal tissue to reshape your eye. The flap goes back into place and, voilá, in a high percentage of cases, the result is corrected vision. Some people are not good candidates for the surgery for reasons related to their vision problem; in most cases the patient is well advised to seek a second opinion from an independent eye doctor (one with no financial ties to the clinic where the surgery would be performed) before going ahead with the procedure.

**Open repair, fractured bone.** In an open repair the surgeon has to cut through skin to gain access to the injured bone, because it has been broken in such a complicated way that it requires the insertion of "hardware" (that is, a screw, plate, rod, or pin) to heal properly. Many different types of anesthesia might be appropriate; it depends largely on what body part needs work. If it's your finger, the doctor might numb just your finger, or perhaps your entire arm, as well as sedate you. If you have a fractured tibia (one of the bones in your lower leg), the surgeon will probably use general anesthesia, or at least an epidural or spinal anesthetic.

**Sinus surgery.** This is surgery done inside your nose (intra-nasally), usually with a scope, to correct a deviated septum, remove bone or bone fragments, or a septum, so that you can breath more comfortably. As in a number of other procedures described here, the choice of anesthesia is strongly influenced by what the surgeon is accustomed to—so if you don't like the doctor's preference, interview other surgeons. Regardless of whether the choice is general or local with sedation, you will be given some numbing medication in your nose. Cocaine-soaked cotton sponges are used in the most common approach, as are drops to prevent bleeding, and/or an injection of a local anesthetic. This part of your body has many blood vessels, so the surgery may cause a lot of bleeding. People with blood pressure problems should be particularly cautious about going ahead with this type of surgery, because rapid blood pressure escalation can result when the doctor uses epinephrine or cocaine sponges to numb the nose.

**Skin lesion removal.** This can be the removal of anything from a benign dot, such as mole or birthmark, to a lesion that's potentially cancerous. It's usually done with local anesthesia, but some surgeons prefer to use a combination of a sedative and a local anesthetic, particularly if the lesion is large. In that case it will usually also be necessary to graft skin to close the area, and the surgeon must get tissue for grafting from another part of your body. Before scheduling your skin lesion removal, I recommend that you find out whether you are likely to need a graft.

**Tonsillectomy.** See "Adenoidectomy."

**TURP (transurethral resection of the prostate).** Men who have benign prostatic hypertrophy (BPH), which means that their prostate is enlarged to a serious degree, will benefit from this procedure. The common symptoms are frequent urination, a feeling of not having voided completely after the urine stream has stopped, and frequent waking at night to urinate. The surgical fix is actually quite simple and not as bad as it sounds. While you are anesthetized with a general, epidural, or spinal, the surgeon inserts a scope through the penis and into the bladder. Using the resectoscope, the surgeon scrapes away at the prostate tissue and removes it through the penis. It comes out in a form that doctors call "prostate chips." If just reading about all this has you covering yourself with protective gestures, then consider asking for a general if your urologist says you need the procedure.

**Tympanoplasty (repair of the eardrum).** This procedure, in which your eardrum is reconstructed, is usually needed when the eardrum doesn't work due to trauma or deformity. The procedure begins with a small incision behind your ear; grafting material is taken from another part of your body, and then it's formed into a substitute eardrum and inserted in your ear cavity. You will need general anesthesia for this surgery, as it usually takes between two to four hours. Nausea, as noted above, can be a significant complication with this surgery, but it can be treated successfully with a ReliefBand, as recommended earlier.

**Varicose vein removal.** Depending on his or her preference, the surgeon can remove your nonfunctioning leg veins in various ways— among them, by laser, scalpel, and sclerosing agents. Small incisions will be made in your leg and the veins will be excised. The numbing can involve sedation with local anesthesia, or general, spinal, or epidural anesthesia. Just be aware that you will need to stand up before surgery so that the blood pools and the surgeon can mark the diseased veins in your legs. Occasionally, anesthesiologists or nurse-anesthetists trying to stay on schedule will give the patient a sedative before the surgeon has had a chance to examine the standing patient to find and mark the veins to be removed. If you're scheduled for this procedure, make sure the marking has been accomplished before you take a sedative.

# Hospital Jargon: A Sample Dialog (with Translation)

When I hear computer geeks throwing around acronyms and technical terms, I understand almost none of what they're saying. I realize that those of us who are medical geeks do the same thing, but people who aren't doctors and nurses might actually want to understand what we're saying, especially since it concerns their well-being. The two scenarios below can help you to get the feel of everyday medical jargon: The first is actually how doctors exchange information; the second is what they would say if they used conventional English.

## IN THE HOSPITAL—MORNING

DR. JONES arrives at 7 AM to relieve DR. SCHWARTZ in the emergency department.

JONES: How was your night?

SCHWARTZ: I got twelve hits.

JONES: Twelve hits! How many players in the ICU?

SCHWARTZ: I have two in ICU.

JONES: Really?

SCHWARTZ: I was gonna send one down to cath lab because his enzymes were bad.

JONES:  No kidding.

SCHWARTZ:  Yeah, he was in CHF. Breathing heavy. He also had COPD, probably from years of smoking.

JONES:  What else did you have?

SCHWARTZ:  I had an MVA.

JONES:  That's a bad night.

SCHWARTZ:  Yeah, he had a pneumo so we put a chest tube in him. Loss of consciousness, too, and his ST waves were off the wall. We had to send him to CAT scan stat.

JONES:  What did it show?

SCHWARTZ:  A whole lot of nothing, except his squash had a subdural hematoma.

JONES:  Who were your other players?

SCHWARTZ:  I had this other guy in ICU that we had to give TPA to right away.

JONES:  How did he do?

SCHWARTZ:  Fine. I was able to turf him to general surgery.

**This is the translation into normal English:**

JONES:  How was your night?

SCHWARTZ:  I got twelve admissions.

JONES:  Twelve admissions! How many patients in the intensive care unit?

SCHWARTZ:  I have two in ICU.

JONES:  Really?

SCHWARTZ:  I was gonna send one down to the catheterization laboratory to have dye injected to outline the coronary arteries and heart structures, because the blood test indicated his enzyme levels were bad.

JONES: No kidding.

SCHWARTZ: Yeah, he was in congestive heart failure. Breathing heavy. He also had chronic obstructive pulmonary disease, probably from years of smoking.

JONES: What else did you have?

SCHWARTZ: I had a patient who'd been in a motor vehicle accident.

JONES: That's a bad night.

SCHWARTZ: Yeah, he had air in the chest wall, so we put a chest tube in him. Loss of consciousness, too, and the waves we saw on his electrocardiogram were off the wall. We had to send him to get a computerized axial tomography scan immediately.

JONES: What did it show?

SCHWARTZ: A whole lot of nothing, except his head had a subdural hematoma.

JONES: Who were your other patients?

SCHWARTZ: I had this other guy in ICU that we had to give tissue plasminogen activator to right away, to dissolve the clots in his coronary arteries.

JONES: How did he do?

SCHWARTZ: Fine. I was able to transfer him to general surgery.

For the definition of other terms not covered in this true-to-life scenario, please check Appendix E, "Glossary of Hospital Terms."

# Useful Websites

## Websites with Good General Directories of Health and Medicine

*dir.hotbot.lycos.com/Health/Medicine*
*dir.yahoo.com/Health*
*www.merckhomeedition.com/home.html*

## Websites of Interest to Patients with a Specific Purpose

### American Board of Medical Specialties (ABMS)
*www.abms.org*
Free Certified Doctor Verification Service allows the public to verify the board certification status, location by city and state and specialty of any physician certified by one or more of the 24 Member Boards of the ABMS.

### Center for Science in the Public Interest
*www.cspinet.org*
Educates about nutrition, alcohol, and many other public health issues.

### Debt Collection Advice over the Internet
*www.lectlaw.com/files/cos26.htm*
If your unpaid hospital bill has been turned over to a debt collection agency, you should know your rights. This website, a free service of

the 'Lectric Law Library, is written in plain English free of legal jargon (as is all the other legal advice for laypersons found on the site—in fact, much of it is written in a colloquial and frequently hilarious style). If you're being harassed by a debt collection agency and want to file a complaint or seek advice from a consumer rights attorney, you can find referrals, plus an interactive Q&A service at: *www.gottrouble.com//legal/finance/debt_collection.html*.

### Dr. Dose, a Service of Mr. Wake-Up
*www.mrwakeup.com*, then click on tab for "Dr. Dose"
Free Internet service that allows you to set reminders to take specific medications at various intervals. You type in the name of the drug you are taking, the times for which you want reminders set, and the telephone number you want called and/or the email address or pager number to which text messages should be sent. Can be customized to suit any medication regimen, no matter how complicated.

### Food and Drug Administration
*www.fda.gov*
In addition to the two websites on food and drug safety listed below, the FDA offers special sections devoted to health issues affecting children, women, and seniors.

Food safety site:
Center for Food Safety and Applied Nutrition
*http://vm.cfsan.fda.gov/list.html*

Drug safety site:
Center for Drug Evaluation and Research
*www.fda.gov/cder/*

### Healthcare Reality Check
*www.hcrc.org*
Science-based information on alternative medicine; features an encyclopedia that links to articles by experts.

### Healthion Corporation
*www.WebMD.com*
A wealth of information, including breaking health care news.

### Healthwire
*www.yourhealth.com*
Health news and online chats with experts.

### HealthWorld Online
*www.Healthy.net*
Helpful tips such as "Calling your Doctor Checklist"—if you can get past the sales aspect of the site.

### International Bibliographic Information on Dietary Supplements
*http://ods.od.nih.gov/databases/ibids.html*
A database of published, international, scientific literature on dietary supplements, including vitamins, minerals, and botanicals.

### Joint Commission on Accreditation of Healthcare Organizations
*www.jcaho.org*
Information also available by telephone: 630-792-5800
The general public section of the site offers guides to help you to select quality health care services.

### KiDz-Med, Inc.
*www.kiDszmed.com*
305-361-6378
Produces a video guide for children who must go to the hospital called *A Hospital Trip with Dr. Bip,* approved by the nonprofit parents' organization, Parents' Choice, 1998, and endorsed by KIDS FIRST!, a project of the Coalition for Quality Children's Media.

### Mayo Clinic Health Oasis
*www.mayohealth.org*
Great information and an excellent search engine leading directly to clearly worded descriptions of diseases, tests, treatment, and articles on key topics such as "What to Expect in the ER."

## Medline Plus Information
*www.nlm.nih.gov/medlineplus/healthtopics.html*
A service of the National Library of Medicine that allows searching through an extensive database of articles from reliable sources.

## Medic Alert Foundation
*www.medicalert.org*
2323 Colorado Avenue
Turlock, CA 95382
888-633-4298
Nonprofit organization that produces Medic Alert bracelets and pendants for persons with conditions such as diabetes, epilepsy, severe asthma, potentially deadly allergic reactions, and other causes of loss of consciousness. In addition to identifying the condition, the Medic Alert tag provides a toll-free number to a monitoring center that retrieves essential medical background information about the tag wearer.

## Medscape
*www.medscape.com*
Sections dedicated to health care professionals and to consumers; the area designed for professionals contains in-depth coverage of new research and a comprehensive database.

## Myvesta.org
*www.myvesta.org*
A nonprofit, Internet-based financial counseling and services organization, offering a free, downloadable publication, "Coping with Medical Bills."

## National Council for Reliable Health Information
*www.ncrhi.org*
Aims to give consumers responsible, reliable, evidence-driven health information; an interesting section called "Hall of Shame" spotlights well-known quacks. Small charge for some literature.

## National Library of Medicine (NLM) of the National Institutes of Health (NIH)
*www.nlm.nih.gov/medlineplus/healthtopics.html*
Covers a broad range of health topics, searchable in a variety of ways. For information about first aid and what to do in an emergency, go to *www.nlm.nih.gov/medlineplus/firstaidemergencies.html*.

## NIH National Center for Complementary and Alternative Medicine
*http://nccam.nih.gov*
The government's own alternative medicine resource; cautions users not to seek the therapies discussed on the site without the consultation of a licensed health care provider.

## Patient Advocate Foundation
*www.patientadvocate.org*
The Patient Advocate Foundation is a nonprofit organization that serves as an active liaison between patients and their insurer, employers, and/or creditors through case managers, doctors, and attorneys to resolve insurance, job discrimination, and/or debt crisis matters related to their diagnosis.

## Public Citizen Health Research Group
*www.citizen.org/hrg/qdsite/orderform.htm*
This nonprofit organization sells publications produced for every region of the United States, with data on doctors who have been disciplined or found guilty of medical malpractice (total in the nationwide database is 20,125). Also offers advice on choosing a safe doctor, improving your quality of medical care, and filing complaints against a doctor.

## Quackwatch
*www.quackwatch.com*
Website of a nonprofit organization dedicated to combating health-related frauds, myths, fads, and fallacies.

## Quicken Family Lawyer
*www.parsonstech.com*
Produces popular program for your computer that guides you through the steps to produce a legally binding document, such as an advance health care directive, a power of attorney for health care, and a will (plus many others on non-health-related issues) in accordance with the laws of your state. Can be ordered and downloaded from the website.

## ReliefBand Device (Woodside Biomedical)
*www.ReliefBand.com*
1915 Aston Avenue
Carlsbad, CA 92008
760-804-6900
fax: 760-804-6925
email: rbinfo@woodsidebiomedical.com
This company produces a wristband that has been found to combat nausea in a wide variety of users, including post-anesthesia patients.

## United States Pharmacopeia
*www.usp.org*
This website furthers the USP's mission of medication error reduction and prevention; provides a helpful page of links to related sites.

## Visiting Nurse Associations of America
*www.vnaa.org*
11 Beacon Street, Suite 910
Boston, MA 02108
617-523-4042
fax: 617-227-4843
email: vnaa@vnaa.org
Helps patients who need in-home nursing care to find qualified caregivers; has links to many other resources for patients at home.

## Web MD
*www.webmd.com*
A good general interest site for the lay reader that gives basic definitions of medical terms and pointers to helpful articles on a wide variety of subjects.

## WellnessWeb
*www.wellweb.com*
Consumer-oriented information with basic explanations of anatomy, diseases, and other health-related topics.

# Glossary of Hospital Terms

For descriptions of common outpatient procedures, see Appendix B.

**3rd-year medical student/4th-year medical student.** In a hospital, a medical student occupies the bottom rung of the authority ladder; his or her badge should state "John/Jane Doe, Medical Student." May be alone when drawing your blood or asking you questions.

**Advance health care directive.** Document with your wishes concerning what may or may not be done on your behalf should you become incompetent to make your own decisions.

**Advanced practice nurse (APN).** A registered nurse with advanced training in a particular area, such as anesthesia practice or midwifery.

**Against medical advice (AMA).** Note put in a patient's chart indicating refusal to accept the doctor's recommendation on a course of treatment.

**Anaphylactic (allergic) reaction.** A series of events in your body triggered by exposure to a specific substance, including the release of chemicals resulting in breathing trouble, hives, or even circulatory arrest.

**Anesthesia care team.** Physician and nurse specialists in anesthesia practice who work on cases together.

**Anesthesia gas analyzer.** A device that analyzes the concentration of inspired anesthetic gas the patient has received; not all hospitals are equipped with it.

**Angiotensin-converting enzyme (ACE) inhibitor.** Medication used to reduce blood pressure by dilating blood vessels.

**Anti-nausea cocktail.** Mixture of three drugs (usually Reglan, Tagamet, and Zofran) that can eliminate nausea and vomiting in most patients; usually must be administered before surgery to be effective. Other, related drugs are available to achieve the same goal.

**Arrhythmia.** Change in the regular beat of the heart, as in, the heart speeds up, slows down, or skips a beat.

**Arthroscopy.** Procedure done with an arthroscope to observe, diagnose, treat, and sometimes repair the interior of a joint—knee, shoulder, ankle, elbow.

**Autologous donation.** Donation of blood by a patient in advance of surgery, to be used by that patient if a blood transfusion is required during surgery; a safety precaution that patients may wish to take in advance of any elective surgery that has the potential for excessive bleeding as a complication.

**Awareness under anesthesia.** Rare occurrence in which the patient under general anesthesia retains the ability to feel pain although can't move or communicate in any way. (See "Bispectral Index System" for information about a means of prevention of such an event.)

**Axillary block.** A type of anesthesia that blocks sensation to your arm by disrupting impulses from major nerves in your armpit.

**Beta-adrenergic block agents (beta-blockers).** Drugs used to treat any of several cardiovascular disorders by slowing the heart rate and lowering blood pressure; also used in migraine therapy.

**Bispectral index system (BIS).** A process for monitoring brain activity to helps anesthesiologists determine whether a patient has awareness during surgery and therefore requires additional anesthesia.

**Blood patch.** See "Epidural blood patch."—An effective treatment of spinal headache, a complication resulting from a leak of spinal fluid caused by the puncture of the needle used to administer spinal or epidural anesthesia; in this treatment, the anesthesiologist repeats the epidural, but the patient's own blood in injected to "patch up the hole."

**Board certification.** Specialty designation earned by a physician after passing specialized written and/or oral examinations.

**Bovie.** See "Electrocautery device."

**Cardiac care unit (CCU).** The intensive care unit for heart patients.

**Cardiovascular technologist/technician.** Medical worker trained to assist your cardiologist in procedures such as angioplasty; monitors your vital signs using electrocardiogram (EKG) and related equipment, and helps to perform other heart-related tests.

**Caudal anesthesia.** Anesthesia that has a localized effect in the lower back, pelvis, and lower extremities; a form of epidural anesthetic.

**Cell saver technology.** A process in which the patient's own blood that otherwise would be lost during surgery is recycled; a sophisticated technology that is not yet available in most hospitals.

**Central venous catheter.** An IV line that can measure the central pressure of the body's venous system.

**Certified nurse-midwife (CNM).** A type of advanced practice nurse who is a registered nurse with advanced training in the management of pregnancy, labor, delivery, and newborn care.

**Certified registered nurse-anesthetist (CRNA).** A type of advanced practice nurse who is a registered nurse with advanced training in anesthesia.

**Chemical code.** Authorization of IV drugs to help save your life, but not electrical intervention, or shock.

**Chemo-receptor trigger zone.** Centers in the brain stimulated by anesthetic medicines or surgical procedures; the area is sensitive to neurotransmitters released during stress and motion, which is why patients prone to seasickness and carsickness are likely to suffer nausea after surgery.

**Chief surgical resident.** Resident in the final year of surgical training.

**Clinical laboratory technologist/technician.** Laboratory worker who examines and analyzes body fluids, tissues, and cells to help doctors diagnose and treat disease; also called medical technologist or technician.

**Clinical nurse specialist (CNS).** A type of advanced practice nurse who is a registered nurse with advanced training and practices in a specialty area.

**Code Blue.** Situation in which the hospital staff pulls out all the stops to save the patient's life—cardiopulmonary resuscitation (CPR), possibly electrical intervention (shocking the patient with a defibrillator), IV drugs, etc.

**Contributory negligence.** In the field of medical malpractice, any action by a plaintiff, such as deliberately ignoring a health practitioner's request to perform a task or follow medical advice that is important to safety or effectiveness of the treatment (for example, not removing jewelry before surgery when requested to do so by hospital staff); in some states a finding of contributory negligence transfers responsibility for any subsequent problem or injury to the patient and absolves the defendant of blame.

**COX-2 (cyclooxygenase-2) inhibitors.** A newer class of anti-inflammatory drugs without many of the side effects of older drugs such as the various NSAIDs (see "Nonsteroidal anti-inflammatory drugs").

**Critical care medicine.** Subspecialty of anesthesiology, surgery, or internal medicine that involves the care of critically ill patients.

**CT scan (computerized tomography).** A sophistical diagnostic tool that forms computerized radiologic images of internal body structures; also called CAT, computerized axial tomography.

**D&C.** Dilatation (sometimes given as "dilation") and curettage; a procedure in which the cervix is dilated and the uterus curetted (scraped out).

**Dantrolene (brand name Dantrium).** The cornerstone therapy for the rare but deadly anesthesia-related condition called malignant hyperthermia (which see).

**Dietitian.** See "Nutritionist."

**Do not resuscitate (DNR) order.** Patient-, family- or guardian-ordered instruction to avert measures to save life; under a DNR order, doctors may administer painkillers such as morphine to make the patient comfortable but will take no "heroic measures" to extend life.

**Doctor of osteopathy (D.O.).** Licensed doctor who trained in a college of osteopathy rather than a medical school that awards the M.D. (doctor of medicine) degree. Although much of the training is identical, osteopaths are taught that the underlying cause of most, if not all, disease is mechanical obstruction in the joints or skeletal system that impedes the flow of the body's natural healing chemicals. Osteopaths study bone and joint manipulation as a "cure" for many types of disease.

**Echocardiographer.** Specialist in tests that diagnose problems with circulation; uses ultrasound instrumentation to collect information such as blood pressure, cerebral circulation, abdominal circulation, and cardiac function.

**Electrocautery device.** Device used to seal (cauterize) blood vessels to stop bleeding; also called a Bovie.

**Electroneuodiagnostic technologist.** Medical assistant who helps physicians diagnose brain disorders, using instruments such as an electroencephalograph (EEG) machine and other measures to assess the effects of infectious diseases or trauma on the brain, and who plays a key role in determining brain death.

**Emergency medical technician (EMT)/paramedic.** Trained medical worker who provides urgent care and transport to a medical facility in the event of serious injury or illness; the life-and-death caregiver dispatched to the scene of an accident or other emergency.

**Emergency department.** See "Emergency room" below.

**Emergency room (ER).** Triage in action; a department of the hospital operating not on the principle of "first come, first served," but of "greatest need, first served." Also may be called "emergency department."

**EMLA cream (eutectic mixture of local anesthetics).** Local anesthetics combined in a white cream; a useful preventive against the pain of an IV stick, for example.

**Endoscopy.** Procedure in which the doctor is able to view a portion of the body with a fiber-optic scope.

**Endotracheal tube.** A breathing tube.

**Epidural anesthesia.** Local anesthesia injected into the back to "freeze" the lower body; the needle is inserted into an expandable space that lies between the skin and the spinal cord (see also "Extradural anesthesia").

**Epidural blood patch.** An effective treatment of spinal headache, a complication resulting from a leak of spinal fluid caused by the puncture of the needle used to administer spinal or epidural anesthesia; in this treatment, the anesthesiologist repeats the epidural, but the patient's own blood in injected to "patch up the hole."

**Epidural catheter.** Tiny plastic tube placed in the epidural space near the nerve roots that emerge from the spinal cord.

**Epidural narcotic administration (ENA).** Metered doses of narcotics administered by a computerized pump over the course of hours or days; the ENA pump infuses the medicine through an epidural catheter into the epidural space.

**Extradural anesthesia.** Local anesthesia injected to the back to "freeze" the lower body; the needle is inserted into an expandable space that lies between the skin and the spinal cord (see also "Epidural anesthesia").

**Family practice.** A medical specialty; the modern equivalent of "the family doctor."

**Fellow.** Doctor in post-residency training who may be training in a subspecialty.

**Fiberoptic scope.** A flexible light source that allows for visualization of internal structures.

**General anesthesia.** Rendering the patient unconscious and insensitive to pain or other surgical stimuli.

**Geriatric medicine.** A subspecialty of family practice or internal medicine that involves care of the elderly.

**GI suite.** Area of the hospital where tests involving the gastrointestinal system are administered.

**Health information technician.** Specialist in keeping health records organized and accessible (what we used to call a "file clerk").

**Health maintenance organization (HMO).** Health care delivery organization in which a particular set of doctors, nurses, and other health care professionals are contractually bound to the medical centers that make up the organization; in theory, HMOs address the total health of their members, but in practice, they may limit patients to only those services and professionals that are part of the organization's network.

**Hospital-based specialty.** Medical practice in fields such as anesthesiology, radiology, pathology, and emergency medicine that is usually performed by doctors under contract to a particular hospital; doctors in these specialties are usually assigned to cases by the hospital, rather than being chosen by the patient.

**House staff.** Doctors, either M.D.s or D.O.s, who work at a particular hospital; at teaching hospitals, includes interns and residents.

**Hypertrophic scar.** Prominent but not painful scarring that is sometimes the result of surgery (see also "Keloid scar").

**ICU psychosis.** See "Sundowning."

**Informed consent.** Doctrine governing your care that implies you have agreed to treatment after you have been informed about the relative benefits and the risks; usually written down in a legal document that the patient is required to sign before surgery or other treatment and diagnostic procedures.

**Inspired anesthesia.** Concentration of anesthetic gas in a patient.

**Intensive care unit (ICU).** Area of the hospital dedicated to acute care of critically ill patients.

**Intensivist.** Specialist in intensive care medicine; the ICU team leader in hospitals that have such a specialist on staff.

**Intern.** First-year post-graduate physician; a doctor who is not yet licensed. Badge might read "Jean Doe—PGY-1," meaning "post-graduate year one."

**Intravenous regional block.** Intravenously administered anesthesia that blocks pain in a particular area of the body, as opposed to the entire body; used in conjunction with a tourniquet to restrict blood flow to and from the affected area.

**Intravenous (IV) lines.** Lines allowing the steady drip of medication, hydrating fluids, or other liquids into the patient's bloodstream, entering a patient's body via a thin plastic tube with a plastic catheter inserted into a vein, often in the hand or arm.

**Intubation.** The placement of a breathing tube in your trachea (windpipe).

**Iodine-based antiseptic.** Rust-colored liquid (Betadine) that protects the patient's skin from infection, but may be caustic to certain skin-sensitive patients, and should be washed off as soon as possible.

**Joint Commission on Accreditation of Healthcare Organizations (JCAHO).** Founded in 1951, an organization dedicated to the improvement of patient safety and quality of care by means of its system of accreditation; the JCAHO evaluates and accredits more than 19,500 health care organizations in the United States.

**July syndrome.** Annual "changing of the guard" in university hospitals after the conclusion of the school year, in which new 3rd-year medical students, interns, residents, and fellows come into the hospital and those of the previous year graduate or rotate out to other departments or hospitals.

**Keloid scars.** Overgrown scars that can burn and itch.

**Licensed practical nurse (LPN).** Medical assistants who receive training in basic nursing skills, including providing direct patient care; their education generally includes a year of hospital and community college courses that focus on the practical aspects of nursing; may or may not be high school graduates. Also known as licensed vocational nurses (LVNs).

**Licensed vocational nurse (LVN).** See "Licensed Practical Nurse"

**Lidocaine.** Local anesthetic with multiple uses in a hospital; also an anti-arrhythmic drug.

**Local anesthesia.** Numbing of a specific part of the body, usually with "-caine" family of drugs (for example, lidocaine, carbocaine, novacaine).

**Magnetic resonance imaging (MRI).** Machine that uses super-powerful magnets to create an image for diagnostic purposes.

**Malignant hyperthermia.** Life-threatening condition, triggered by certain anesthetics and characterized by high fever and hyper-metabolism; predisposition to it is inherited (see "Dantrolene").

**Mammographer.** Medical technician who makes images of breast tissue used in diagnosing breast diseases, especially breast cancer.

**Medical record technician.** See "Health information technician."

**Medical toxicology.** A subspecialty of preventive medicine; the study of substances toxic to humans.

**Migraine equivalent.** Migraine episode not in the form of a headache. A migraine can come in the form of other symptoms and signs; it can mimic a stroke, severe abdominal pain, and more.

**Narcotic.** Powerful painkiller; the family of drugs includes Demerol, codeine, Percodan, and many others. Common side effects include urinary retention, nausea and vomiting, itching, constipation, and difficulty breathing.

**Naso-gastric (NG) tube.** Tube that runs from the nose down to the stomach through which a patient may be fed or have stomach contents suctioned out.

**National Practitioner Data Bank (NPDB).** Created by an act of Congress in 1990, the NPDB keeps track of physicians who have been disciplined by medical boards or professional societies, paid on malpractice suits, and/or had hospital privileges suspended for more than 30 days. Although access is restricted to medical professionals, members of the public can find much of the same information published in region-by-region directories of "Questionable Doctors" produced the nonprofit organization, Public Citizen Health Research Group (on the Internet at *www.citizen.org/hrg/qdsite/orderform.htm*).

**Nerve block.** Type of anesthesia involving the numbing of nerves, typically in the arm or leg, but also face or torso.

**Nitrous oxide.** Inhaled anesthetic gas used to supplement general anesthesia; also known as "laughing gas."

**No Code Blue.** Opposite of "Code Blue," a situation in which heroic interventions will not be taken to save the patient's life; same as "do not resuscitate" order.

**Nonsteroidal anti-inflammatory drug (NSAID).** Class of drugs including many common medications such as aspirin, Naprosyn, and

Advil; NSAIDs usually do not cause the side effects of narcotics, but can be associated with ulceration, bleeding, and kidney damage.

**Nuclear medicine.** Area of the hospital where diseases are diagnosed using radionuclides, unstable atoms that spontaneously emit radiation.

**Nuclear medicine technologist.** Medical assistant who administers a radioactive tracer, then operates cameras that detect and map the tracer to detect abnormalities.

**Nurse-practitioner (NP).** A type of advanced practice nurse; NPs have diagnostic skills, manage therapy by outlining care, sometimes provide prescriptions, coordinate consultations and referrals, and counsel on lifestyle changes that promote good health.

**Nurse's aide.** A hospital worker with limited medical training, who usually performs routine patient care chores under the supervision of a registered nurse; usually has very limited formal medical education. See also "Unlicensed assistive personnel (UAP)."

**Nutritionist.** An expert in meal planning and nutrition programs who supervises the preparation and serving of meals in the hospital; sometimes called "Dietitian/Nutritionist."

**Occupational medicine.** A subspecialty of preventive medicine focused on occupational issues.

**Occupational therapist.** Therapist who assists people who have been impaired in some way to regain normal functioning or learn adaptive techniques in order to perform the daily tasks of life.

**Operating room technician/technologist.** A medical assistant who helps set up the operating room with surgical instruments and equipment, sterile linens, and sterile solutions; may perform other key tasks associated with the OR, including passing instruments and other sterile supplies to surgeons and surgeon assistants and preparing patients for surgery; may also be responsible for OR cleanup.

**Patient-controlled analgesia (PCA).** Anesthesia delivery device designed for patients staying overnight in the hospital; the PCA pump responds to a patient's command (usually by the push of a button) to send a dose of a painkilling drug or drug combination into the IV line and then to the bloodstream.

**Patient advocate.** A person on the hospital staff, or consulting with the hospital, charged with representing the patient about various rights, especially when the patient is incapacitated or for other reasons cannot argue forcefully on his or her own behalf; the term is also used for a person chosen by the patient—usually a close relative or friend—who has agreed to look after that patient's interests and help out with personal needs during the patient's hospital stay.

**Pharmacist.** A trained professional who is licensed to dispense drugs prescribed by a doctor and can give advice about those drugs to consumers.

**Phlebotomist.** Clinical laboratory technician who draws the patient's blood.

**Physical therapist (PT).** Therapist who uses exercise, physical manipulation, and related treatments to help patients needing rehabilitation from injury or disease.

**Physician's assistant (PA).** Medical assistant trained to perform a range of tasks previously only performed by doctors, including history taking, physical exam, diagnosis, and patient management; often the primary source of care in remote areas.

**Plastic closure.** Also known as a subcuticular stitch, a method of closing a wound, commonly used by plastic surgeons because the result is usually cosmetically more appealing than other closures.

**Preventive medicine.** A medical specialty focused on averting medical problems in particular environments.

**Progress notes.** Daily written assessment of a patient's hospital progress, also called a SOAP note, that is, Subjective (patient's complaint), Objective (doctor's observation), Assessment, and Plan.

**Propofol.** Anesthetic drug that has grown in popularity because, among other things, it can result in pleasant dreams for the patient and have a significant anti-nausea effect; on the downside, it's suspended in an egg-soy-lecithin emulsion, so a true egg allergy might elicit an adverse reaction to this drug.

**Pulse-oximeter.** A device clipped around the patient's pulse, usually to a finger or a toe, that monitors the patient's heartbeat and measures the amount of oxygen in the blood.

**Radiographer.** Another term for an X-ray technician (see "Radiologic technologist").

**Radiologic technologist.** Medical assistant who uses diagnostic imaging equipment to record the condition of the patient's internal organs and bones.

**Radiology.** Medical specialty and area of hospital focused on diagnostic images such as X-ray, CT scan (see above) and MRI (see above).

**Raynaud's disease.** Interrupted blood flow to the extremities (finger and toes, and sometimes the ears and nose) caused by exposure to cold; often linked to some other health problem, such as lupus, rheumatoid arthritis, or other autoimmune disease.

**Recreational therapist.** Therapist who addresses the patient's physical, mental, and emotional well-being through activities such as games, dancing and music; also known as a "therapeutic recreation specialist."

**Regional anesthesia/block.** Anesthesia affecting an isolated body part, usually not as limited in area as a local anesthetic.

**Registered nurse (RN).** Person who has completed a state-approved education program in patient care and passed a licensing examination; 60 percent of RNs work in hospitals, where they monitor and coordinate patients' daily care.

**Resident.** Doctor starting formal training in a specialty such as internal medicine, anesthesiology, obstetrics, or any of several dozen others.

**Respiratory therapist.** Therapist who evaluates, treats, and cares for patients with breathing disorders; respiratory therapists treat all types of patients, ranging from newborns whose lungs are underdeveloped to older people whose lungs are diseased.

**Rounds.** Daily route through the hospital of doctors and doctors in training, in which patients' cases are reviewed and discussed in practical and theoretical terms.

**Sedation.** Commonly known as "twilight anesthesia," a state of semi-consciousness, usually induced with narcotics, sedatives, or both.

**Self-donation of blood.** See "Autologous donation."

**Sensitivity.** A negative response to a substance, but not involving the chemical responses associated with an allergy (See "Anaphylactic reaction").

**Sodium citrate.** Inexpensive, salty-tart liquid that reduces stomach acid.

**Sonogram.** The use of sound waves to create an image of internal body structures. Also called "ultrasound."

**Speech-language pathologist/audiologist.** Medical assistant who works with people who can't speak normally or with patients who have oral motor problems causing eating and swallowing difficulties; audiologist focuses on hearing, balance, and related problems.

**Spinal anesthesia.** Local anesthesia applied to the patient's back to "freeze" the lower part of the body; works well for many procedures that involve only the lower part of the body.

**Spinal headache (post-dural puncture headache).** Potential side effect of both spinal and epidural anesthesia that results when the needle punctures the fluid-filled sac surrounding the brain, the spinal cord, and its branches; the leak of spinal fluid leads to headaches when the patient is sitting or standing up.

**Subcuticular stitch.** See "Plastic closure."

**Subspecialist.** A doctor who is board-certified in a specialty and has passed additional tests to earn certification in a more specific area of practice, for example, pediatric cardiology (focused on children with heart problems), which is a subspecialty of cardiology.

**Succinylcholine.** Muscle relaxant commonly used in anesthesia with surgical patients.

**Sundowning.** Phenomenon that occurs most typically in the early evening, in which a patient becomes disoriented, disengaged from reality, agitated, and even combative; also called ICU psychosis.

**Surgical technologist.** See "Operating room technologist/technician."

**Teaching hospital.** Not necessarily just a medical center at a university, but any hospital, public or private, that accept medical students, interns, residents, and fellows, and provides them with an educational experience in affiliation with a medical college or university program.

**Telemedicine.** Use of computer, imaging, and communications equipment to close the geographic gap between those who have a medical need and those who have the expertise to help them.

**Tertiary care hospital.** Major hospital center integrating patient care, research, and teaching.

**Topical anesthesia.** Anesthesia applied directly to skin, mucous membranes, or cornea, usually in the form of liquid, gel, or cream.

**Triage.** French for "sorting"; in the context of a hospital emergency room, a method by which doctors and nurses establish the priority of medical treatment for each patient in need of treatment.

**Ultrasound.** See "Sonogram."

**Unlicensed assistive personnel (UAP).** Another term for nurse's aides, who may or may not have received any formal training in nursing skills in an educational institution.

**University hospital.** Teaching hospital associated with a university.

**Urinary catheter.** Thin tube that allows urine to drain from the bladder.

**Walking epidural.** Form of epidural anesthesia involving a lower concentration of the local anesthetic so that the patient can still walk around during the process of labor.

**X-ray technician.** See "Radiographer" and "Radiologic technologist."

# ACKNOWLEDGMENTS

## From David Sherer

I would like to thank the many professionals who helped make this book come about. I appreciate the work of my copy editor Patricia Borthwick, as well as designer Cindy Peters. Special thanks go out to Jo Ellen Murphy for her clever and creative cover designs. Also thanks to Peggy Robin for her editorial input and fresh ideas. Finally, a big thank you to all the doctors, nurses, technicians, assorted medical personel and patients who have contributed their experiences and wisdom.

## From Maryann Karinch

My sincere thanks go to Bill Adler and Peggy Robin for their contributions of expertise and guidance; to my agent, Laura Belt, whose keen insights help every project; to my constant sources of information and inspiration, my partner, Jim McCormick and my mother, Ann; and to Jim's mother, Mary Helen, whose positive experiences with medical professionals helped shape some of the book's content. I also thank all of the friends and acquaintances who gave us input that helped shape the recommendations and stories.

3rd-year medical student 5-6, 206, 281
4th-year medical student 206, 281
    *See also* medical students
Acid blocker 134-135, 65
Acid reflux 65, 62
Advance health care directive 104-107, 281
Advanced practice nurse (APN) 218, 281
African Americans and scarring 61
Against medical advice (AMA) 110, 281
Alcohol 46
Alcohol, and anesthesia 83, 131-132
Allergy 46, 47-48, 52, 85-86, 183, 281
Alternative medicine 92
    *See also* herbal supplements
Alternative physical therapy 250
Ambulance 179-180
American Board of Medical Specialties (ABMS) 10
Anabolic steroids 67
Analgesic drugs, and side effects 92
    *See also* Narcotics, NSAIDS, and COX-2
Anaphylactic (allergic) reaction 47-48, 281
Anesthesia, and allergies and sensitivities 85-86
Anesthesia, and informed consent 109-110
Anesthesia, and medical history 79-86
Anesthesia, and nausea 87-88, 140
Anesthesia care team 71, 79, 80, 282
Anesthesia gas analyzer 282
Anesthesia monitor 80, 86

Angiotensin-converting enzyme (ACE) inhibitor 282
Anti-arrhythmic drug 88
Anti-nausea cocktail 88, 282
Anxiety and surgery 58, 141
Arrhythmia 282
Arthroscopy 282
Artificial implants, and surgery 57
Asthma 63, 157, 183
Asthma inhaler 66, 134
Attending physician 143, 208, 210
Autologous donation 62, 282
    *See* self-donation of blood
Awareness under anesthesia 86, 282
Axillary block 73, 282
Battery 111
Beta-adrenergic block agents (beta-blockers) 283
Bispectral index system (BIS) 86, 283
Blood patch 283
Board certification 10-11, 79, 283
Body piercing, and surgery 138-139
Bovie 57, 138, 283
Call button 161
Cardiac care unit (CCU) 239, 240, 283
Cardiovascular technologist/technician 230, 283
Cast 160-161
Catheter 61, 72, 146, 226
Caudal anesthesia 72, 283
Cell saver technology 62, 283
Central venous catheter 61, 283
Certified Doctor Verification Service 10
Certified nurse-midwife (CNM) 218, 221, 284
Certified registered nurse-anesthetist (CRNA) 79, 88, 218, 221
Cesarean section (C-section) 135
Chemical Code 105, 284
Chemoreceptor trigger zone 87, 284
Chief surgical resident 207-208, 284
Clinical laboratory technologist/technician 230, 284
Clinical nurse specialist (CNS) 220-221, 284
Code Blue 105, 284
Community Hospital 31-32, 34, 38-39
Contact lenses, and surgery 139

Contributory negligence 284-285
Corticosteroids 63, 66-67
COX-2 (cyclooxygenase-2) inhibitors 92, 285
Critical care medicine 285
CT scan (computerized tomography) 285
D&C 285
Dantrolene 86-87, 285
Dental injury, and anesthesia 81
Dentures, and surgery 139
Diabetes 63, 66, 128, 183
Dietary Supplement Health and Education Act (DSHEA) 53
Dietary Supplement Poison Center Study Group (DSPCSG) 57
Dietary supplements 85
    *See also* Herbal supplements
Dietitian 228, 232-233, 285
Discharge instructions 241-242, 246
Do not resuscitate (DNR) order 104, 285
Doctor of Osteopathy (D.O.) 213, 285-286
Driving after surgery 248-249
Drugs, and adverse reactions 46, 49-51, 82-83, 150
Drugs, and allergies 46-47, 52, 153-154,
Drugs, and brand names 250
Drugs, and children 171
Drugs, and current prescriptions 48
Drugs, and dietary supplements 53-56
Drugs, and race 51
Drugs, and reporting on pre-surgical questionnaire 48, 49-50
Drugs, and sensitivities 47-48, 52, 153-154
Drugs, and surgery 65-67
Eating before surgery 60, 131, 132
Echocardiographer 230, 286
Elective surgery 5,8,62, 136
Electrocautery device 138, 286
    *See also* Bovie
Electroneurodiagnostic technologist 230-231, 286
Emergency contact information 96, 121, 185, 201
Emergency medical technician (EMT)/paramedic 184-185, 188-190,
    196-198, 286
Emergency Medical Treatment and Labor Act 181
Emergency room (ER) 177-179, 186-198, 203, 286
Emergency room care team 195

Emergency room, and children 187
Emergency room, and health insurance 180-181
Emergency room, and personal items 201-202
Emergency room physician 196
EMLA cream (eutectic mixture of local anesthetics) 170-171, 286
Endoscopy 286
Endotracheal tube 145-146, 287
Ephedra (ma huang) 54, 85
Epidural anesthesia 72, 74, 75, 76-77, 132-133, 147, 149, 287
Epidural blood patch 148-149
Epidural catheter 90, 287
Epidural narcotic administration (ENA) 89-90, 91, 287
Epilepsy 62, 65, 183
Extradural anesthesia 287
Family health history 43, 45, 84
Family practice 219, 287
Fellow 206, 208, 287
Fiberoptic scope 287
First aid kit 198
Food and Drug Administration, U.S. (FDA) 53
Gastroesophageal reflux disease (GERD) 62, 135, 183
Gene related drug reaction 50-51
General anesthesia 61, 72, 76-77, 86, 145, 287
General anesthesia, and children 166-168
General hospital 31, 34, 36
Geriatric medicine 288
Ginko 54
Ginger 150
Ginseng 54
GI suite 288
Harassment 215-216
Health information technician 288
Health insurance company representative 95, 101
Health insurance coverage 28, 99-102, 247, 254
Health insurance, and exclusion 99-103
Health insurance, and travel 200-201
Health maintenance organization (HMO) 9, 78, 221, 224, 288
Herbal supplements 53-56, 85, 245-246
Home care 246-247, 248
Home care, and medical equipment 249-250
Hospital accreditation 28-30

Hospital-based specialty 78, 288

Hospital caused infections, and prevention 144

Hospital food 128-129, 158

Hospital policies, and children 168

Hospital ratings 30-31

Hospital room 115-118, 157

Hospital stay, and current prescriptions 121

Hospital stay, and dress 132

Hospital stay, and entertainment 123-128, 235

Hospital stay, and packing 118-124, 126

Hospital stay, and packing for children 169-170, 173

Hospital stay, and religious preferences 154-156, 158

Hospital stay, and storage of personal items 123-124, 201-202

Hospital tour 35, 116

Hospital tour, and children 38-39, 165-166

Hospital types

    *See* community, general, religiously affiliated, and teaching hospitals

House staff 212, 213-215, 288

    *See also* fellows, interns, and residents

Hypertrophic scar 61, 288

Informed consent 107-110, 288

Informed consent, and children 166-167

Inhaled anesthesia 86

Insomnia 65

Inspired anesthesia 289

Insulin, and surgery 66

Intensive care unit (ICU) 52, 239-240, 289

Intensive care unit (ICU) psychosis 158-159

Intensivist 240, 289

Intern 6, 37-38, 143-144, 206-207, 211-212, 214, 289

Internet 20-21, 217

    *See also* Appendix D "Useful Websites"

Intravenous regional block 289

Intravenous (IV) start 171, 226

Intubation 63, 80, 183-184, 289

Iodine-based antiseptic 289

IV lines 56, 88, 90, 146

Jewelry, and surgery 138

Joint condition 63, 67

Joint Commission on Accreditation of Healthcare Organizations
  (JCAHO) 28-29, 251, 253, 289

July syndrome 5-8, 289-290
Kava 54
Keloids 61, 290
Ketamine 78
Latex allergy 56
Licensed practical nurse (LPN) 221-222, 225
Licensed vocational nurse (LVN) 221-222, 225
Lidocaine 88, 170, 290
Local anesthesia 73, 74-75, 76-77, 88, 90, 141, 290
Magnetic resonance imaging (MRI) 57, 234, 235, 290
Make-up and surgery 137-138
Malignant hyperthermia 84, 86-87, 290
Malpractice 103, 108, 112, 251-252
Malpractice criteria 110-11
Mammographer 290
Mask, and anesthesia 166
Medical bills 103-104, 253-255
Medical history 43-46, 62, 79-86, 182-183
    *See also* family health history
Medic Alert Foundation 183-184
Medical education, and philosophy 213
Medical emergency identification card 257-258
Medical alert bracelet 183-184
Medical questionnaire 43, 44-45, 48
Medical record technician 6, 290
Medical students 5-7, 32, 37-38, 143-144, 206-207, 211, 213
    *See also* 3rd year medical students and 4th year medical students
Medical toxicology 290
Medication
    *See* drugs
Medication card 181-182
Medication schedule 242-243
Melaleuca oil 54
Migraine equivalent 291
Nail polish, and surgery 138
Narcotic 83, 92, 149, 243, 291
Naso-gastric (NG) tube 61, 146, 226, 291
National Practitioner Data Bank (NPDB) 111-112, 291
Nerve block anesthesia 72, 73, 76-77, 291
Nitrous oxide 78
No Code Blue 105, 291

Non-surgical alternatives 24-25
Nondrug pain control 92
Nondrug therapy 159-160
Nonsteroidal anti-inflammatory drugs (NSAIDs) 92, 153-154, 291-292
Nuclear medicine 231, 292
Nuclear medicine technologist 231, 292
Nurse-practitioner (NP) 218, 219, 220, 224-225, 292
Nurse's Aide 222, 225-226, 292
Nutritionist 228, 232-233, 285, 292
Obesity 63-64
Obesity, and intubation 63
Occupational medicine 292
Occupational therapist (OT) 228, 233, 292
Organ donation 106
Operating room technician 292-293
Outpatient procedures 259-268
Oxygen mask, and anesthesia 89
Pacemaker, and surgery 66
Patient-controlled analgesia (PCA) 89, 90, 91, 92, 293
Patient advocate 7, 95-100, 103, 145, 150, 151, 159, 174-175,
    208, 251, 293
Patient Advocate Foundation 99
Patient rights 2-3, 7-8, 150, 208
Pediatric Hospital 187
Penicillin 153, 183
Pharmacist 293
Phlebotomist 239, 293
Physical therapist (PT) 228, 233, 293
Physician's assistant (PA) 219-220, 224-225, 293
Plastic closure 61, 293
Post-dural puncture headache
    *See* spinal headache
Post-operative pain control 89-90, 149-150
Power of attorney for health care 106
Pre-surgical questionnaire 43-44, 46, 48
Pre-surgical instructions 60
Preventive medicine 46, 294
Primary care physician 9, 10, 11, 107, 185-186
Privacy 35, 37, 45, 162
Private doctor 208, 213-214, 216
Progress notes 294

Propofol 52, 72-73, 294
Public Citizen Health Research Group 30, 112-113
Pulse-oximeter 63, 294
Radiographer 294
Radiologic technologist, 231, 294
Radiology 234
Raynaud's disease 63, 294
Recovery room, and children 168-169
Recreational therapist 229, 233, 294
Referral 9-12, 79, 233
Refuse treatment, right to 7
Regional anesthesia/block 73, 76-77, 295
    *See also* epidural, spinal, local, and nerve block
Registered nurse (RN) 78, 218, 222-223, 225-227, 295
ReliefBand 87, 140
Religiously affiliated hospital 32-33, 34, 36, 118
Resident 6, 37-38, 143-144, 207-208, 214
Respiratory therapist 229, 295
Rounds 212, 295
Same sex caregiver 154-156
Scar 61, 290
Second opinion 16, 17-18
Sedation 72, 75, 78, 83, 133, 295
Sedation, and children 167
Self-donation of blood 62, 295
    *See also* autologous donation
Senior physician 208
Sensitivity 47-48, 85-86, 295
Shaving, and surgery 133
Skin cream, and surgery 137
Skin sensitivities 56-57, 143
Sleep apnea, and intubation 64-65, 80
Smoking, and surgery 46, 133-134
Social services worker 246
Sodium citrate 135, 295
Sonogram 295
Specialized hospital 32, 34, 36, 37
Speech-language pathologist/audiologist 229, 233, 295-296
Spinal anesthesia 72, 73-74, 76-77, 147, 296
Spinal headache 147-149, 296
St. John's wort 54, 85

Stomach acid 135
Subcuticular stitch 61
    *See* plastic closure
Subspecialist 10, 14, 296
Substance abuse and anesthesia 84
Succinylcholine 84-85, 86, 296
Sundowning 158-159, 296
Support groups 22-23
Surgeon, and experience 7, 8, 15-16, 58-59, 211
Surgeon, and selecting 9-20, 14-15
Surgery, and scheduling 5, 6, 8, 9, 59-60
Surgical technician/technologist 232, 296
Surgical wound 160
Sutures 61
Teaching hospital 7-8, 32, 34, 37-38, 143-144, 205-206, 210, 247, 296
Telemedicine 217, 297
Tertiary care hospital 297
TMJ and intubation 80
Topical anesthesia 72, 297
    *See also* EMLA
Transportation to and from hospital 125-126, 179-180, 187
Triage 186, 297
Triage nurse 196
Ultrasound
    *See* Sonogram
University hospital 5-6, 8, 205-206, 297
Unlicensed assistive personnel (UAP) 222, 225-226, 297
    *See also* nurse's aide
Urinary catheter 61, 297
Valium 76, 78
Visiting hours 39, 129-130, 173-174
Visiting Nurses Association 246
Walking epidural 297
Wills 104
X-ray technician 231, 234

# ABOUT THE AUTHORS

*Dr. David Sherer* was born in Washington, DC, and grew up in Bethesda, Maryland. After earning a BA in music from Emory University, he went on to medical school at Boston University and trained in anesthesia at the University of Miami. To date, he has anesthetized some 30,000 surgical patients, and has lectured to professional medical and nursing groups. He is the holder of two US patents for medical and communications devices, and has acted in television commercials. An avid runner, he lives in Chevy Chase, Maryland, with his wife Laura and son Liam. He has learned a lot from his father, Max, who is in his fifty-third year of active medical practice.

*Maryann Karinch* has written about medicine, technology and fitness for 25 years and published seven books. She lives in Half Moon Bay, California. Her website is ***www.karinch.com***.